EAT YOUR AGE

EAT YOUR AGE

Feel Younger, Be Happier,

Live Longer

IAN K. SMITH, M.D.

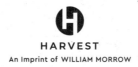

HARVEST

An Imprint of WILLIAM MORROW

This book contains advice and information relating to health care. It should be used to supplement rather than replace the advice of your doctor or another trained health professional. If you know or suspect you have a health problem, it is recommended that you seek your physician's advice before embarking on any medical program or treatment. All efforts have been made to assure the accuracy of the information contained in this book as of the date of publication. This publisher and the author disclaim liability for any medical outcomes that may occur as a result of applying the methods suggested in this book.

The material on linked sites referenced in this book is the author's own. Harper-Collins disclaims all liability that may result from the use of the material contained at those sites. All such material is supplemental and not part of the book. The author reserves the right to operate or close the website in his sole discretion following December 2024.

FIRST EDITION

Library of Congress Cataloging-in-Publication Data has been applied for.

ISBN 978-0-06-338355-5

25 26 27 28 29 LBC 6 5 4 3 2

CONTENTS

A NOTE FROM THE AUTHOR

There's been a wonderful shift in the attitudes of many when it comes to health, appearance, and longevity. Yes, people still want to lose weight. Yes, people still want to look good on the beach during vacation. Yes, people still want that attention from friends and strangers when they walk into a room. There's nothing wrong with these desires, and it's unlikely there will ever be a time when they are not somewhere on the priority list. But many are now looking at these snapshot moments as being part of a more holistic view of want they want in life. They want to not only live longer, but also live better. People understand that natural aging is a natural part of life, but they are also aware that a decent portion of *how* they age is within their grasp.

I have always been fascinated with the body and what it takes to keep it looking and feeling good and functioning well. Why must we resign ourselves to more weight around the midsection or the inability to climb two flights of stairs without getting winded simply because we've added another year on our birthday calendar? What's so magical about the age of 40, 50, or 60 that mandates you no longer play the sport or participate in the hobbies you've enjoyed for most of your life? The answer to both questions is that you absolutely are not obligated to give up on these activities that you've enjoyed for so long simply because the clock is ticking. There's so much you can do to keep yourself looking and feeling youthful, and it doesn't depend on how much money you have or how many times you visit the plastic surgeon. It's about how well you plan, how aware you are of your body and health, and the simple steps you can take to forge a path of vigor and vitality that has nothing to do with the number of candles on your birthday cake. *Eat Your Age* is your travel guide, a road map of sorts, of easy and doable measures and information-gathering that you can undertake right away to make your years not only long but incredibly strong, filled with purpose, great memories, and an abundance of sheer joy.

Ian K. Smith, M.D.

1

DEFY AGE

For hundreds of years, there have been fabulous stories of rulers and explorers looking for the fountain of youth—magical water that could bestow the restorative powers of youthful vigor to those who drank or bathed in it. It has been rumored that Alexander the Great encountered a healing "river of paradise" in the fourth century BCE. But this legend is not the only one. From Japan to England to the Canary Islands, mythical tales of magical healing and miracles were rampant. Despite the tremendous effort put forth and the power of those commissioning this enviable search for infinite youth, success was elusive. That was then, and this is now. Maybe the intentions of their search weren't as misguided as the locations they were searching and the form in which they were expecting to find this source of abundant youth.

Today, there are numerous stories of people who have found some form of that youthful fountain. It wasn't the water they drank or the river they swam in, rather it was what they ate, how they moved, and their philosophical approach to life. The headlines and viral video clips populate the media. "75-year-old Charles Allie Goes Sub-14 in the 100m at Penn Relays." "World's Oldest Female Bodybuilder, 86, Can Still Bench 50kg and Lives Off Nuts and Eggs." "World's Oldest Ironman Plans to Keep Competing into His 90s." The subjects of these headlines, Charlie Allie, Ernestine Shepherd, and Hiromu Inada are the living embodiments of defying age. They, along with many other older competitors, have amazed the world with their physical performances, conquering challenges that adults a quarter their age have not even tried, let alone succeeded in doing. Instantly, reading their stories and watching their videos makes you wonder aloud, "How is this even possible?" But it also begs the question, are these exceedingly rare accomplishments and performances a signal that the fountain of youth has finally been found? The answer will vary based on what definition you decide to use.

It's extremely unlikely without some revolutionary scientific achievement that humans will be able to live for hundreds of years and enjoy almost eternal youth. But maybe the scaled-back version of this is what we're seeing with the previously mentioned athletes as well as the scores of centenarians around the world who are not just reaching ages that were once thought unachievable but are also maintaining a relatively good quality of life and participating in vigorous activities.

Our perception of aging typically centers around gray hair, wrinkled, sagging skin, hunched shoulders, curved spine, shuffling gait, and emaciated extremities. We think of older people sitting and chatting on a park bench, being pushed in a wheelchair to a doctor's appointment, or walking cautiously with a cane as others pass them by. We don't think about people in their 80s racing, participating in bodybuilding competitions, or conquering an IRONMAN triathlon that consists of a 2.4-mile swim, 112-mile bicycle ride, and 26.2-mile run. This traditional thinking that aging automatically means a dramatic change in appearance and steep decline in function can and should be changed by taking small, early steps that can keep you feeling and looking young longer.

If you want to know how to grow old without feeling old, why not learn from those who have done it? *National Geographic* Fellow Dan Buettner along with Michel Poulain and Giovanni Mario Pes have done extensive and highly informative research in this field. They studied regions all over the world called Blue Zones that produce the most centenarians and focused on the specific aspects of their lifestyle and their living environments that contributed to their longevity. Their research, along with that conducted by others, has created a treasure trove of information that can be instructive for those looking for the modern version of the fountain of youth.

This entire book is dedicated to helping you find ways to prevent, combat, and slow the typical physical, mental, and spiritual decline of aging. I'll provide specifics on how this is done in the coming chapters, but below you will find the general strategic framework of 15 things that you can implement in your life at any age to immediately start turning back the clock—or at least prevent it from running out too quickly.

Ingredients for a Recipe to Glorious Aging

1. Find purpose.
2. Stay hydrated.
3. Cut back on salt.
4. Protect your skin.
5. Exercise your heart.
6. Limit alcohol.
7. Sleep long and deeply.
8. Exercise your brain.
9. Visit your dentist.
10. Eat more plants, less meat.
11. Stress less.
12. Find your community.
13. Increase vitamin C intake.
14. Gorge on antioxidants.
15. Fill up on fermented foods.

Find purpose. Living just to be living and doing just to be doing might get you through the day or week or month, but it won't serve you in the long run. Having purpose, whatever that might mean to you, gives you focus and creates intentionality in what you do. Having a definable "why" is something that many people who live long and well have in common. There is no fixed list of what "whys" are most effective. This is something that's organic and you must own. Ask yourself why you're getting out of bed every morning, and if your answer is not one of fulfillment or that generates a sense of usefulness, then it's time to think harder about your direction. Researchers have long expounded that purposeful living—whether it be increasing social activity, reducing stress, or treating depression—can be the spark for good health and longevity. Find what it is in life that makes it all worth it and cling to it tightly, holding it up as your North Star.

Ways to Lead a Purposeful Life

- Discover your passions and pursue them.
- Live in the present and experience moments fully.
- Have and express gratitude for even the small things.
- Identify your values and try to follow them.
- Form meaningful relationships.
- Empower others.
- Set goals that help define your path.
- Contribute to and support your community.

Stay hydrated. Most people who are walking around dehydrated don't even realize it. We are constantly losing water from our body and it's not just when we go to the bathroom. Sweating and breathing also play big roles in how we diminish our important supply of H_2O. Not only is our body about 60 percent water, but we need it for many important bodily processes, including carrying nutrients to our cells, lubricating and cushioning our joints, maintaining a normal body temperature, protecting our spinal cord and other sensitive tissues, and eliminating wastes when going to the bathroom. Consuming sufficient quantities of water throughout the day is critical, even when we're not sweating. Remember, you are losing water all the time, and to maintain optimal health, you need to replace it to maintain proper levels in our body.

Cut back on salt. High-sodium foods can lead to a bevy of health problems, including high blood pressure, heart disease, and stroke. Too much salt can also erode that youthful appearance. High levels of sodium cause the body to retain water, and when this happens in your face, you can develop a puffier appearance that can be particularly noticeable under your eyes. According to the Harvard School of Public Health, most Americans consume at least 1.5 teaspoons of salt per day, which is the equivalent of about 3400 mg of sodium—more than double what most people need. Surprisingly, most of the sodium we eat is not the salt we sprinkle on our food at the table, rather, it's already present in the packaged foods we consume. The next time you go shopping, turn over the package, can, or bottle and look at the nutrition label. Check out the line listed for sodium and up top at the number of servings contained in the package. Remember, that amount you're reading is *per* serving, so if it says 30 mg and there are three servings in the package, that means the total package contains 90 mg of sodium. It's important to know the numbers as they can directly impact your health.

Protect your skin. The sun doesn't just feel good on the skin, it also helps activate vitamin D, which is crucial to our health, especially our bones. However, too much sunlight can wreak havoc on our skin. There is a fine line between what is healthy and what is unhealthy. There are no hard time guidelines for what is considered enough or too much, but generally, the key is to avoid burning. Most people can stay in the sun for up to an hour during peak sun (between 10 a.m. and 2 p.m.) without burning. But for some, that amount of time might be only a matter of minutes based on your sun sensitivity and how much sun protection you have on from sunscreen, clothing, sunglasses, and hats. Years of unprotected exposure to the sun takes a heavy toll that you don't notice while you're young and enjoying the bronzing of your skin. But as you get older, it's time to pay the bill, and your body reflects this in sagging, wrinkling, and uneven, spotty skin that can look aged and unhealthy. Using sunblock and sunscreen can help protect your skin from skin cancer, prevent early aging, and keep it looking young for a long time.

Exercise your heart. The four chambers that beat every second of your life deep inside of your chest are the most important muscles in your body. Without them functioning properly, your health can be severely compromised. Heart disease is the number one killer in the world and for good reason. It can creep up on you, and when you finally receive a diagnosis, it can be too late to reverse a lot of the damage that's already been done. Regular exercise or physical activity is the key to keep your heart beating strong and long. Just like the muscles in your legs and arms need to be regularly trained to remain strong and viable, so too does your heart. It's fine to do steady-state exercises in which the workout is a continuous, steady effort. However, dynamic exercises in which the intensity of your energy output varies might prove more beneficial. You can take something that is typically steady state, like walking, and convert it to a dynamic exercise by changing the pace and topography of where you're working out. If you're on a treadmill, change the speed and incline. If you're outside, walk on different surfaces and vary the pace of your walk. Get your heart rate higher for several minutes, then let it slow down before returning it to a faster pace. Walk a course that's not always flat but has some inclines and declines. They don't have to be dramatic, but something that provides some challenge. This variation is good training for one of your body's most vital organs.

How to Measure Your Heart Rate

1. Using the pads/tips of your index (pointer) and middle fingers, press them gently against the side of your neck (just under your jawline). Or . . .
2. Using the tips of your index and middle fingers, press on the inside of your wrist, below the base of your thumb.
3. Count the number of beats you feel for 15 seconds. Use a stopwatch or other timing device to track the seconds accurately.
4. Multiply the number of beats by 4.
5. That number is your heart rate.

For example, if you count 22 beats in 15 seconds, multiply 22 by 4, for a total of 88 beats per minute.

Source: Mass General Brigham Hospitals

Limit alcohol. Alcohol is one of those things where some is fine, but too much can be a bad thing. The health benefits of red wine and its powerful antioxidants such as resveratrol and proanthocyanidins have been well researched and documented. One or two glasses can keep the balance on the healthy side; however, too much can tip into the unhealthy zone. Excessive alcohol consumption can lead to damage of the liver and contribute to chronic health conditions such as high blood pressure, diminished immune system responses, cancer, mental health challenges, and unintentional injuries (falls, drowning, motor vehicle accidents, burns, and firearm injuries). The Centers for Disease Control and Prevention (CDC) recommends one drink or less per day for women and two drinks or less per day for men. This recommendation is based on body size, which can help determine how well the alcohol is handled (metabolized) by the body. Remember, it's not the type of alcohol you drink that matters most, rather, it's the amount of alcohol consumed that most affects your health.

Sleep long and deeply. Sleep might be the most underrated part of the day for many. The attitude that if extra time is needed to accomplish things throughout the day, you can just borrow it from your sleep hours is ill-advised. Imagine driving your car on a ten-hour trip, then once you reach your destination, you park it, and instead of turning off the engine you keep it running overnight. That's effectively what you're doing when you are up all day tending to life's activities, then you go to sleep for just a few hours and get back up and enter the busy fray of life again. Your body's engine needs rest and time to restore. Numerous studies have looked at the impact of poor sleep on health and found that not only can it cause problems with learning, focusing, and reacting, but sleep deprivation can put you at higher risk for cardiovascular disease and early death. What's the magic sleep number? There's no universal consensus, but most sleep experts believe it's at least seven hours per night. People living in the Blue Zones are typically getting eight to ten hours, and in some places, afternoon naps are a regular part of the day. Adequate sleep is not a luxury but a necessity for good health.

Dr. Ian's Tip

BLACKOUT BLUE LIGHT

Millions of people suffer from sleep deprivation or poor sleep quality. In some cases, there are medical reasons such as obstructive sleep apnea that are the cause. However, for many people, it's their environment that's the root of the problem. Our devices have become some of the biggest culprits of sleep disruption. Blue light from our devices seems to be the most disruptive light at night as it's believed to suppress the secretion of melatonin, a hormone necessary for good sleep. This suppression can shift the body's circadian rhythm, which is our biological clock, and this can send a signal to the brain to wake up instead of slow down. Studies have shown that even a few hours of exposure to blue light at night can slow or stop the release of the sleep hormone melatonin. Bottom line, try to avoid looking at bright screens at least two hours before going to sleep and you might feel better rested the next morning.

Exercise your brain. While your brain is not anatomically categorized as a muscle, it certainly behaves like one. Challenging it and using it to perform higher function tasks as well as engaging in physical exercise can be important for growing new nerve cells (neurons) and nerve connections (synapses), making new neuronal pathways, and maintaining peak performance. There's an old adage that if you don't use your brain, it will turn to mush. Well, it might not physically disintegrate into a bowl of soup, but certainly it's functioning might begin to resemble such. Participating in brain-stimulating activities on a regular basis (such as learning a new language, playing memory or video games, working on puzzles such as crosswords, jigsaws, or number problems, playing board games, learning a musical instrument) pays dividends as it can prevent or slow the process of dementia, keep your memory sharp, and keep you more deeply engaged in your activities, environment, social relationships, and life in general.

Visit your dentist. We often think that visiting our dentist is either a luxury or should be done only in a time of emergency. Nothing can be further from the truth. Regular dental visits are critical to monitor the health of your teeth. Just like diseases that affect other parts of the body, catching oral conditions early can be critical in implementing treatment that can rectify the problem and prevent further damage. It's also important to know that health problems in other parts of the body might first appear in your mouth. A regular checkup could make you aware of other medical issues that are brewing and need to be addressed before too much damage is done. Visit your dentist for an exam at least once a year, and while you're there, make sure you get a thorough teeth cleaning.

Eat more plants, less meat. The potential health impact of eating too much red meat is well documented. Similarly, the benefits of eating a more plant-based diet have been well researched and widely recommended by leading health experts throughout the world. When looking at the Blue Zones of the healthiest, longest-living people on earth, researchers found that the residents were not strict vegetarians; however, while they did eat some meat, it was infrequent and in much smaller portions. Their diets largely consisted of whole grains, legumes, garden vegetables and herbs, and foods rich in unsaturated fats such as avocados, nuts, fish, seeds (flax, pumpkin, sesame) and oils (canola, corn, flaxseed, olive, peanut, soybean, and sunflower). Remember, saturated fat is unhealthy, and unsaturated fat is healthy. Numerous studies from all over the world have examined the dietary habits of thousands of people from Japan to Greece and the research consistently shows that a plant-based diet leads to less health problems and a longer and healthier life.

Stress less. All of us, regardless of our education level, financial status, gender, age, or any other attribute will experience stress at some point in our lives. In fact, some degree of stress is a good thing. It can condition us to handle future challenges more efficiently and effectively so that we are able to function and survive during times of high stress. This is what is called the fight-or-flight response that humans exhibit when confronted with a potentially traumatic, high-stakes situation. However, stress that is too severe or too persistent can become a problem. Chronic stress can speed up the aging process in many ways. There are decades' worth of research that have connected and documented the relationship between stress and mental health. There is also evidence that stress can affect us beyond mental health, as it can be a risk factor for autoimmune disease, cancer, heart disease, and neurological diseases.[1] Scientists have wondered what could be happening at the molecular level that's causing this potential impact. Yale University researchers looked at this question and found that stress can affect our microscopic DNA.[2] They looked at the human biological clock, something that governs all of us and represents patterns of chemical changes our DNA goes through as we age. It's believed that these stress-related changes to our biological clock accelerate the aging process, which leads to a shorter life. While you can't always control the person, event, or circumstances producing the stress, there are things you can do to mitigate its impact. The Yale study found that people who had strong emotional regulation and self-control skills had younger biological clocks than those who didn't possess these attributes. Other stress relievers that have been found to be beneficial involve simple things such as walking outside, deep breathing, resting, meditation, praying, listening to music, and gardening. There are many ways to blunt the deleterious impacts of stress, so find whatever works best for you and add it to your tool kit.

Find your community. There are times when you might want to be alone and enjoy the simplicity of being in a controlled environment where you can dictate your interactions with others. Getting away can be an opportunity to recharge and reconsider your life's perspectives. But there is definitely something to the concept of finding and building community and healthy social relationships. Blue Zone research from Ogliastra in Sardinia found that strong family and community connections were an integral part of people's lives. Elders were looked after by the younger members, while there was plenty of assistance offered to help raise each other's children. Researchers reported seeing residents, even on what most of us consider to be business-only workdays, gathering to laugh and play games throughout the town. These findings are not surprising as other research has shown that people with strong social support networks have a lower risk of developing cardiovascular diseases such as heart attacks and strokes. These social connections have even been linked to decreased levels of inflammation in the body and improved immune function, which can help slow the aging process. Find your community, take your mind off the stressors in life, and enjoy a sense of belonging and purpose.

Increase vitamin C intake. The potential benefits of vitamin C are widespread—it can boost immunity, protect memory, prevent iron deficiency, fight inflammation, and lower the risk for heart disease. Vitamin C also can play an important role in how your skin ages, so it's important to make sure you are consuming sufficient amounts in the foods that you eat or supplements you take. While this important vitamin is commonly found in many foods such as citrus, broccoli, peppers, and berries, as well as various over-the-counter supplements, it can also be found in a topical formulation, which can be applied to the skin. It provides several benefits, including slowing the signs of aging, preventing sun damage, and reducing the blemishes of dark spots, acne, and wrinkles. Topical vitamin C should be in your skin hygiene arsenal to keep your skin looking young, tight, and invigorated.

Gorge on antioxidants. Antioxidants are tiny compounds that can be found in a variety of fruits and vegetables that protect the cells against free radicals—molecules that can lead to damage that results in health problems such as heart disease and cancer. Eating more plant-based foods will help you load up on these sturdy disease fighters which also include vitamin E and a group of antioxidants called carotenoids (found in tomatoes, carrots, orange bell peppers, corn). Some of the foods with the highest amounts of antioxidants are red beans, berries (blueberries, blackberries, raspberries, strawberries), pinto beans, apples, plums, and dark leafy greens.

Fill up on fermented foods. According to the National Center for Biotechnology Information, fermented foods are defined as those foods or beverages produced through controlled microbial growth, and the conversion of food components through enzymatic action. Basically, these are foods and drinks that contain live microscopic bacteria, yeast, or fungi. You might know these organisms by the more popular name probiotics. It's highly likely that you've been eating these foods and didn't even know they were part of the fermented family. They include aged/raw cheeses, kefir, kimchi, kombucha, miso, natto, pickles, sauerkraut, sourdough bread, tempeh, and yogurt. Fermented foods have anti-inflammatory and antioxidant properties that are good for your gut; they help with digestion, boost your immune system, and help maintain the proper diversity of good and bad bacteria inside of your body (microbiome). There are also beauty products that are made with fermented extracts that some dermatologists believe can help calm and brighten the skin.

Now you have your list of 15 simple, affordable things you can add to your life's routine that can have an immediate impact on the quality and length of your life. In the following chapters you will learn the specifics of what you need to do and know depending on your current age. The goal is that once you finish the last chapter, you will be able to develop a customized road map that will help you navigate this wild and unpredictable adventure we call life, thus putting you in prime position to squeeze every ounce of goodness and optimal health out of it.

The Inspiration

Camille, a 73-year-old retired schoolteacher, had always led a relatively healthy lifestyle, but as she entered her

70s, she began experiencing health issues typical of aging, such as arthritis, hypertension, and decreased mobility. Concerned about her declining health, Camille sought advice from her doctor, who emphasized the importance of lifestyle changes in managing her conditions and improving overall health. She and her doctor created a plan and went to work.

The Plan

Diet modification: Camille didn't become a vegetarian, but she adopted a more plant-based diet rich in fruits, vegetables, whole grains, and lean proteins. She minimized processed foods, sugar, and saturated fats, opting instead for nutrient-dense meals that supported her overall health and provided essential vitamins and minerals.

Regular exercise: Despite her arthritis, Camille incorporated gentle exercises into her daily routine, such as walking, swimming, and yoga. With guidance from a physical therapist, she developed a personalized exercise plan that focused on improving flexibility, strength, and balance.

Stress reduction techniques: Recognizing the impact of stress on her health, Camille practiced mindfulness meditation, deep breathing exercises, and relaxation techniques. By managing stress more effectively, she experienced improved sleep quality and reduced symptoms of anxiety and depression.

Social engagement: Camille prioritized social connections by participating in community activities, volunteering at local organizations, and joining senior groups. These social interactions provided emotional support, companionship, and a sense of belonging, which contributed to her overall well-being.

The Change

Over the course of several months, Camille's dedication to lifestyle behavior changes yielded remarkable results.

1. She achieved a healthy weight through her improved diet and regular exercise regimen, reducing the strain on her joints and improving her mobility.
2. By adopting a low-sodium diet and engaging in regular physical activity, she successfully lowered her blood pressure, reducing her risk of cardiovascular complications.
3. She experienced a noticeable increase in energy levels and overall vitality, allowing her to participate more fully in daily activities and pursue her interests with enthusiasm.
4. Through stress reduction techniques and social engagement, she reported a significant improvement in her mood, mental clarity, and overall emotional well-being.

Camille's inspiring journey exemplifies the transformative power of lifestyle behavior changes in defying age and optimizing health in later life. By prioritizing nutrition, exercise, stress management, and social connections, she not only improved her physical health but also enhanced her quality of life and embraced aging with vitality and resilience. Her story serves as a testament to the importance of proactive self-care and the limitless potential for growth and rejuvenation at any age.

2

KNOW YOUR
HIDDEN DANGERS

The journey of aging is mirrored by the journey of our health. Our bodies are in a constant state of evolution as we age, making it imperative that we are equipped with knowledge to live our best and healthiest life. Some might view the aging process as walking through a field of mines of varying sizes and destructive potential. It's virtually impossible not to step on some of the mines, but the hope is to do it as infrequently as possible and to make sure the mines that are eventually contacted are the smallest and least destructive. This chapter is aimed at helping you navigate the health minefield so that you can live the highest quality of life with the fewest health challenges for the longest time possible.

As we age and our bodies change based on genetics and the environments we subject ourselves to, our risks for certain diseases and conditions rise and fall. There are certain conditions, such as cystic fibrosis or febrile seizures, that are largely and almost exclusively diagnosed in the young. There are conditions such as Alzheimer's and osteoarthritis that are most commonly diagnosed in our later years. Our risk for certain health conditions is a complicated interplay between genetics, environment, and lifestyle behaviors. For example, fair-skinned people who are exposed to unobstructed sunlight for prolonged periods of time are at greater risk for devel-

MEDICAL DANGERS PER DECADE

30S	40S	50S	60S+
Anxiety	Anxiety	Anxiety	Alzheimer's Disease
Bone Calcium Loss (W)	Breast Cancer	Breast Cancer	Breast Cancer
Cervical Cancer (W)	Depression	Depression	Cataracts
Depression	Diabetes (Type 2)	Diabetes (Type 2)	Chronic Obstructive Pulmonary Disease (COPD)
Diabetes (Type 2)	Erectile Dysfunction (men)	Heart Disease	Colorectal Cancer
High Cholesterol	Muscle Loss	High Cholesterol	Dementia
Infertility	Obesity	Hypertension (high blood pressure)	Diabetes (Type 2)
Iron Deficiency	Overactive Bladder	Muscle Loss	Heart Disease
Muscle Loss	Perimenopause (women)	Osteoarthritis	High Cholesterol
Prediabetes		Osteoporosis	Hypertension (high blood pressure)
Sleep Disorders			Muscle Loss
Testicular Cancer (M)			Osteoarthritis
			Parkinson's Disease
			Rheumatoid Arthritis

oping skin cancer. A woman who has family members with a history of breast cancer due to mutated versions of the BRCA1 and BRAC2 genes has a significantly increased chance of carrying the same mutation and, according to the American Cancer Society, her risk of developing breast cancer by the age of 80 is an astounding seven out of ten.

Knowledge is power, and that is particularly relevant when it comes to knowing and understanding what conditions are most common during different decades of life. This knowledge is vital, because it gives us the opportunity to take preventive measures to either avoid these conditions altogether or catch the conditions in their earlier stages when they can be promptly treated and/or cured before too much damage is done. For example, look at hypertension (high blood pressure), which, according to the National Institutes of Health (NIH), is the leading cause of cardiovascular disease and premature death not just in the United States, but worldwide. While hypertension is sometimes diagnosed in adults as young as 30, it is most commonly diagnosed in adults in their 60s and 70s. This means that starting in your 30s, you should start thinking about what risk factors you need to avoid or modify so that as you get closer to the peak age range for hypertension, you have greatly reduced your chances of developing this severely debilitating and potentially lethal condition.

This chapter will help you better understand what those lurking hidden medical dangers are that correlate to your current decade of life and those medical conditions you are more likely to face later in life. A person in their 30s should not only be concerned about the most common health conditions that afflict their decade, but they should also look at other decades to learn what might be coming and what they can do to prevent or slow its emergence. At the end of the chapter, you will find brief definitions/descriptions of all the medical conditions that have been indicated for the various decades.

In the table below, you will find the various conditions and the signs and symptoms that characterize them. Find the conditions that

CONDITION AND SIGNS AND SYMPTOMS

Alzheimer's Disease

Symptoms can vary from person to person, but here are some common signs and symptoms of early stage Alzheimer's Disease:

- Confusion around dates or current location
- Constantly losing things or misplacing them in odd places
- Difficulty completing otherwise simple tasks
- Difficulty handling money and paying bills
- Forgetting recently learned information
- Increased anxiety and/or aggression
- Taking longer to complete normal daily tasks
- Loss of spontaneity and initiative
- Memory loss that disrupts daily life
- Planning or problem-solving becomes difficult
- Exhibiting poor judgment that leads to poor decision making
- Wandering and getting lost

Anxiety

- Difficulty concentrating
- Difficulty controlling feelings of worry
- Easily fatigued
- Increase in headaches, muscle aches, stomach aches, or unexplained pains
- Irritability
- Sleep problems (difficulty falling asleep or staying asleep)

Bone Calcium Loss (women)

There are no signs and symptoms until a severe enough stage has been reached. Consuming adequate amounts of calcium is critical during this decade.

Breast Cancer

- Any change in size or shape of the breast
- New lump in the breast or armpit
- Nipple discharge, including blood
- Pain in any location of the breast
- Pulling in of the nipple or pain in the nipple area
- Redness or flaky skin in the nipple area or other parts of the breast
- Thickening or swelling of part of the breast

Cataracts

- Eye color looks faded
- Difficulty seeing well at night or in low light
- Double vision (sometimes goes away as cataracts get larger)
- Lamps, sunlight, or headlights seem too bright
- Seeing halos around lights
- Vision is cloudy or blurry

Cervical Cancer (women)

Early Stage

- Pelvic pain or pain during sex
- Vaginal bleeding after sex
- Vaginal bleeding between periods or periods are heavier or longer than normal
- Vaginal discharge that's watery and has a foul odor.

Chronic Obstructive Pulmonary Disease (COPD)

- Chest tightness
- Chronic cough that may produce mucus that might be clear, greenish, yellow, or white
- Frequent respiratory infections
- Lack of energy
- Shortness of breath/difficulty breathing during physical activities
- Unintended weight loss (advanced stages)
- Wheezing

Dementia

- Difficulty performing complex tasks
- Difficulty planning and organizing
- Increasing confusion
- Loss of ability to do everyday tasks
- Memory problems
- Personality or behavior changes
- Poor coordination and control of movements
- Problems communicating or finding words
- Problems with reasoning or problem-solving
- Reduced ability to concentrate
- Unexplained apathy/depression/withdrawal

Depression

According to the National Institute of Mental Health, if you have been experiencing some of the following signs and symptoms, most of the day, nearly every day, for at least two weeks, you may be experiencing depression:

- Changes in appetite or unplanned weight changes
- Decreased energy, fatigue, or feeling slowed down
- Difficulty concentrating, remembering, or making decisions
- Difficulty sleeping, waking early in the morning, or oversleeping
- Feelings of guilt, worthlessness, or helplessness
- Feelings of hopelessness or pessimism
- Feelings of irritability, frustration, or restlessness
- Persistent sad, anxious, or "empty" mood
- Physical aches or pains, headaches, cramps, or digestive problems that don't have a clear physical cause and don't go away with treatment

Diabetes (Type 2)

- Blurred or decreased vision
- Dark patches of skin around the armpit, neck, or groin
- Dry mouth
- Frequent unexplained fatigue
- Frequent urination
- Impotence or erectile dysfunction
- Increased hunger
- Increased thirst
- Irritability
- Numbness/tingling in hands or feet
- Slow-healing sores
- Unintended weight loss

Erectile Dysfunction (men)

- Reduced sexual desire
- Inability to get an erection
- The ability to get an erection sometimes, but not every time you want to engage in sex
- The ability to get an erection, but it's not sustained long enough to engage in sex

Heart Disease

Sometimes heart disease can be "silent" and undiagnosed until a person experiences signs or symptoms of a heart attack. Symptoms can also depend on the type of heart disease one has.

Congenital Heart Defects

- Pale gray skin or lips (cyanosis)
- Swelling in belly area, legs, or around the eyes

Congestive Heart Failure

- Cough that doesn't go away or brings up white or pink mucus with spots of blood
- Difficulty concentrating or decreased alertness
- Fatigue and weakness
- Rapid or irregular heartbeat (arrhythmia)
- Rapid weight gain from fluid buildup
- Reduced ability to exercise
- Shortness of breath or difficulty breathing while lying down
- Swelling in legs, ankles, and feet
- Wheezing

Coronary Artery Disease

- Chest pain, discomfort, pressure, and tightness
- Pain in the jaw, neck, throat, upper abdomen, or back
- Pain, numbness, weakness, or coldness in the arms or legs
- Shortness of breath

Irregular Heartbeat

- Chest pain or discomfort
- Dizziness
- Fainting (syncope) or near fainting
- Fluttering in the chest
- Lightheadedness
- Racing heartbeat (tachycardia)
- Shortness of breath
- Slow heartbeat (bradycardia)

Valvular Disease

- Chest pain
- Fainting
- Fatigue
- Irregular heartbeat

- Shortness of breath
- Swollen feet or ankles

High Cholesterol

There are no symptoms. This condition can only be detected through a blood test.

Hypertension (High Blood Pressure)

This is a dangerous disease because it typically has no warning signs or symptoms, and many people don't even know they have it. This is why it's called the "silent killer." Measuring your blood pressure is the only way to know if you have high blood pressure.

Those who have very high blood pressure might experience some symptoms such as:

- Abnormal heart rhythm
- Anxiety
- Blurred vision or other vision changes
- Buzzing in the ears
- Chest pain
- Confusion
- Difficulty breathing
- Dizziness
- Nausea
- Nosebleeds
- Severe headaches
- Vomiting

Infertility (men and women)

Women

- Inability to get pregnant
- Menstrual cycle that's too long (35 days or more)
- Menstrual cycle that's too short (less than 21 days)
- Menstrual cycle that's irregular or absent
- Painful periods that might include back pain, pelvic pain, and severe cramping

Men

Symptoms can be vague or nonexistent. Sometimes, an underlying problem causes signs and symptoms.

- Abnormal breast growth (gynecomastia)
- Changes in hair growth

- Changes in sexual desire
- Decreased facial or body hair
- Difficulty with erections and ejaculation
- Inability to conceive a child
- Inability to smell
- Lower than normal sperm count
- Pain, lump, or swelling in testicles
- Recurrent respiratory infections
- Testicles that are small and firm

Iron Deficiency (women)

- Brittle nails
- Chest pain, fast heartbeat, or shortness of breath
- Cold hands and feet
- Extreme fatigue without an identifiable cause
- Headache, dizziness, or light-headedness, especially with activity
- Pale skin (or yellow)
- Pounding or "whooshing" in the ears
- Tongue inflammation or soreness or smoothness
- Unusual cravings for nonnutritive substances such as ice, dirt, or starch
- Weakness that's generalized and unexplained

Muscle Loss

- One arm or leg smaller than the other
- Difficulty lifting items that could previously be lifted
- Numbness or tingling in arms and/or legs
- Weakness in an arm or leg

Obesity

- Check your BMI and waist circumference.

Your body mass index can be found in any online BMI chart or BMI calculator. Your waist circumference is the measurement taken around the abdomen at the level of your belly button. Measure with a soft tape measure.

Osteoporosis

Called a "silent" disease, because typically there are no symptoms until a bone is broken. Some potential symptoms before significant fracture occurs include:

- Back pain
- Loss of height over time
- Stooped posture

Overactive Bladder

- Frequent urination (for many this could mean more than eight times in 24 hours)
- Urgency: strong urge to urinate that you can't ignore
- Leaking urine when you feel the sudden urge to go
- Waking up at night more than once to go to the bathroom

Parkinson's Disease

- Impaired posture, balance, and coordination
- Loss of automatic movements such as blinking, smiling, or arm swinging while walking
- Muscle stiffness where the muscles remain in a contracted state for a long time
- Slowed movement
- Speech changes such as speaking softly or quickly, slurring, or hesitation
- Tremor usually beginning in a limb, often the hand or fingers
- Writing changes in which writing becomes difficult and might appear small

Prediabetes

Doesn't usually have any signs or symptoms, however, one possible sign is darkened skin on certain parts of the body (armpits, groin, neck).

Rheumatoid Arthritis

- Morning stiffness that goes away as the day progresses
- Pain and stiffness that worsens with inactivity and improves as the joint is warmed up with increased activity
- Pain, stiffness, and swelling in one or more joints
- Reduced range of motion about the joint

Sleep Disorders

There are many types of sleep disorders. However, most can be characterized by the presence of one or more of the symptoms below:

- Difficulty falling or remaining asleep
- Difficulty staying awake during the day
- Irregular or insufficient sleep

- Prone to unusual behaviors (abnormal movements, talk, emotions, and actions like sleepwalking) that disrupt sleep

Testicular Cancer (men)

Some men have no symptoms at all. Many of the symptoms below are more likely to be caused by something other than testicular cancer but can also be seen in those with the disease:

- Back pain
- Breast growth or soreness
- Dull ache in the lower belly or groin
- Early puberty
- Feeling of heaviness in the scrotum
- Lump or swelling in either testicle
- Pain or discomfort in a testicle or scrotum
- Sudden swelling in the scrotum

commonly affect your decade in the table above, then use the table below to familiarize yourself with those signs and symptoms so that in the event you experience any, you can seek advice from a healthcare professional as soon as possible.

Self-awareness is the first step in treating any of these conditions and preventing further complications. The phrase "knowledge is power" might be a cliché, but its relevance in maintaining and restoring good health can't be overstated. Knowing the health challenges you are likely to encounter and the early signs and symptoms to watch out for can be critical to your leading a better-quality and happier life. While it can be extremely helpful to learn and understand about these conditions and the signs and symptoms that go along with them, it's still critical that you consult with a qualified healthcare professional who can properly diagnose your condition and develop a plan of action if one is needed. Don't delay seeking help since early intervention can be crucial to preventing the worsening of your condition. Below you will find brief descriptions of these conditions. Speak to your healthcare provider for more in-depth information and consultation.

ALZHEIMER'S DISEASE

Alzheimer's disease is a debilitating neurodegenerative disorder characterized by progressive cognitive decline, primarily affecting memory, thinking abilities, and behavior. It is the most common cause of dementia, accounting for around 60 to 70 percent of dementia cases. The disease typically begins with subtle memory lapses, such as forgetting recent conversations or events, and progresses over time to more severe impairment, including difficulty with language, reasoning, and problem-solving skills. As Alzheimer's advances, individuals may experience confusion, disorientation, mood swings, and changes in personality and behavior. Activities of daily living become increasingly challenging, eventually leading to a loss of independence.

Alzheimer's disease is associated with the accumulation of abnormal protein deposits in the brain, including beta-amyloid plaques and tau tangles, which disrupt communication between nerve cells and contribute to cell death. The exact cause of this protein aggregation is not fully understood, but it is thought to involve a complex interplay of genetic, environmental, and lifestyle factors.

Risk factors for Alzheimer's disease include age, family history, certain genetic mutations, cardiovascular disease, diabetes, and a history of head injuries. While advancing age is the greatest known risk factor, Alzheimer's is not a normal part of aging.

ANXIETY

Anxiety disorders encompass a range of mental health conditions characterized by persistent feelings of fear, worry, or nervousness that are disproportionate to the actual threat or situation. These feelings can be overwhelming and interfere with daily functioning, affecting various aspects of life, including work, relationships, and personal well-being. There are several types of anxiety disorders, each with its own specific symptoms and triggers:

Generalized anxiety disorder (GAD): People with GAD experience excessive worry and anxiety about a wide range of everyday concerns, such as health, finances, work, or relationships. This worry is often difficult to control and may be accompanied by physical symptoms like restlessness, fatigue, muscle tension, and difficulty concentrating.

Panic disorder: Panic disorder is characterized by recurrent panic attacks, which are sudden episodes of intense fear or discomfort that reach a peak within minutes. Panic attacks can be accompanied by physical symptoms such as heart palpitations, sweating, trembling, shortness of breath, and a sense of impending doom or loss of control. People with panic disorder often live in fear of experiencing another attack and may avoid situations or places where they fear an attack could occur.

Social anxiety disorder (social phobia): Social anxiety disorder involves an intense fear of social or performance situations where the person may be scrutinized or judged by others. This fear can lead to avoidance of social gatherings, speaking in public, or participating in activities where they may feel exposed. Physical symptoms may include blushing, sweating, trembling, nausea, or difficulty speaking.

Specific phobias: Specific phobias are irrational fears of specific objects, situations, or activities. Common phobias include fear of heights (acrophobia), fear of spiders (arachnophobia), fear of flying (aviophobia), or fear of enclosed spaces (claustrophobia). When confronted with their phobic trigger, individuals may experience intense anxiety or panic.

Anxiety disorders can have various causes, including genetic factors, brain chemistry, environmental stressors, and traumatic experiences.

Treatment for anxiety disorders typically involves a combination of therapy, medication, and self-care strategies. Cognitive-behavioral therapy (CBT) is often used to help individuals identify and challenge negative thought patterns and develop coping skills to manage anxiety. Medications such as selective serotonin reuptake inhibitors (SSRIs), serotonin-norepinephrine reuptake inhibitors (SNRIs), or benzodiazepines may be prescribed to alleviate symptoms.

BONE CALCIUM LOSS

Bone calcium refers to the mineral calcium stored within the structure of bones. Calcium is a crucial mineral for the formation, growth, and maintenance of bones. About 99 percent of the body's calcium is found in bones and teeth, where it provides strength and rigidity. Bone calcium plays several vital roles in the body:

Bone structure: Calcium gives bones their hardness and strength, contributing to their structural integrity.

Bone formation: During bone growth and development, calcium is essential for the mineralization process, where calcium salts are deposited into the collagen matrix, forming hard bone tissue.

Bone remodeling: Throughout life, bone tissue undergoes continuous remodeling, with old bone being resorbed by osteoclasts and new bone being formed by osteoblasts. Calcium is required for both processes.

Muscle contraction: Calcium ions are released from bones into the bloodstream when needed for muscle contraction and other physiological processes. This dynamic equilibrium helps regulate calcium levels in the blood.

Nerve function: Calcium ions are involved in transmitting nerve impulses and regulating various cellular processes.

Maintaining appropriate levels of bone calcium is crucial for overall health. Insufficient calcium intake can lead to weakened bones, increasing the risk of fractures and osteoporosis, while excess calcium can contribute to kidney stones or other health issues. Regular weight-bearing exercise and a balanced diet rich in calcium and vitamin D are essential for maintaining healthy bone calcium levels.

BREAST CANCER

Breast cancer is a complex disease characterized by the uncontrolled growth and division of abnormal cells in the breast tissue. It can originate from different parts of the breast, including the ducts that carry milk to the nipple (ductal carcinoma) or the glands that produce milk (lobular carcinoma). In some cases, it can also develop in the connective tissues or other cells within the breast.

Risk factors for breast cancer include genetic factors, such as mutations in genes like BRCA1 and BRCA2, which significantly increase the likelihood of developing the disease. Other risk factors include increasing age, hormonal factors (such as early menstruation or late menopause), a personal or family history of breast cancer, dense breast tissue, radiation exposure, obesity, alcohol consumption, and hormone replacement therapy.

Breast cancer can manifest with various symptoms, although some individuals may not experience any noticeable signs initially. Common symptoms include a lump or mass in the breast or underarm area, changes in breast size or shape, dimpling or puckering of the skin, nipple discharge (other than breast milk), nipple inversion or retraction, redness or scaling of the skin on the breast or nipple, and persistent breast pain.

Early detection is crucial for improving treatment outcomes and survival rates. Screening methods such as mammography, clinical breast exams, and breast self-exams can aid in detecting breast cancer at an early stage when it's most treatable. Mammograms, in particular, can identify abnormalities in the breast tissue before they become palpable.

The treatment for breast cancer depends on various factors, including the type and stage of the cancer, as well as the individual's overall health and preferences. Treatment modalities may include surgery (such as lumpectomy or mastectomy), radiation therapy, chemotherapy, hormone therapy (to block hormones that fuel cancer growth), targeted therapy (which attacks specific molecules involved in cancer growth), or a combination of these approaches. Regular follow-up care and adherence to recommended screening guidelines are essential for monitoring and managing the disease effectively.

CATARACTS

Cataracts are a common eye condition characterized by the clouding of the natural lens inside the eye, leading to blurred vision. This clouding typically develops gradually over time and can vary in severity, eventually interfering with daily activities such as reading, driving, or recognizing faces. While aging is the primary cause of cataracts, other factors such as genetics, prolonged exposure to ultraviolet light, certain medical conditions like diabetes, use of corticosteroid medications, and eye injuries or surgeries can also contribute to their development. Symptoms may include blurry vision, faded colors, increased sensitivity to glare, difficulty seeing at night, and frequent changes in eyeglass or contact lens prescriptions. Cataracts can often be effectively treated through surgery, during which the clouded lens is removed and replaced with an artificial one, restoring clear vision.

CERVICAL CANCER

Cervical cancer is a malignant disease that originates in the cells of the cervix, the narrow passage connecting the uterus to the vagina. Most cases of cervical cancer are caused by persistent infection with certain types of human papillomavirus (HPV), a sexually transmitted infection. Over time, HPV infection can lead to the development of abnormal cells in the lining of the cervix, which, if left untreated, can progress to cervical cancer.

Cervical cancer typically progresses slowly, starting with precancerous changes known as cervical dysplasia or cervical intraepithelial neoplasia (CIN). If these abnormal cells are not detected and treated, they can eventually develop into invasive cancer, spreading beyond the cervix to nearby tissues and organs.

Preventive measures such as HPV vaccination, practicing safe sex, and undergoing routine cervical cancer screening are crucial for reducing the risk of developing cervical cancer and improving outcomes for those affected by the disease. Once diagnosed, treatment options for cervical cancer may include surgery, radiation therapy, chemotherapy, or a combination of these approaches, depending on the stage and characteristics of the cancer.

CHRONIC OBSTRUCTIVE PULMONARY DISEASE (COPD)

Chronic obstructive pulmonary disease (COPD) is a chronic inflammatory lung disease that causes obstructed airflow from the lungs. The primary symptoms include difficulty breathing, cough, and excessive mucus production. The two most common forms of COPD are chronic bronchitis and emphysema.

Chronic bronchitis: In chronic bronchitis, the airways that carry air to the lungs (bronchial tubes) become inflamed and produce excess mucus, leading to cough and difficulty breathing.

Emphysema: Emphysema involves the destruction of the air sacs (alveoli) in the lungs, which reduces the surface area available for gas exchange. This results in difficulty in breathing and decreased oxygenation of the blood.

Cigarette smoking is the leading cause of COPD, although long-term exposure to other lung irritants, such as air pollution, chemical fumes, or dust, can also contribute to its development. COPD is a progressive disease, meaning it worsens over time, and it can significantly impact a person's quality of life. Treatment often involves medications to manage symptoms, such as bronchodilators and corticosteroids, as well as lifestyle changes like quitting smoking and pulmonary rehabilitation programs to improve lung function and overall well-being. In severe cases, supplemental oxygen therapy or surgery may be necessary.

DEMENTIA

Dementia is a broad term that is used to describe a range of symptoms related to a decline in cognitive function (thinking, remembering, and reasoning) that interferes with a person's daily life and activities. It is not a specific disease but rather a syndrome characterized by a progressive loss of cognitive abilities. There are many different causes of dementia, with Alzheimer's disease being the most common. Other causes include vascular dementia, Lewy body dementia, frontotemporal dementia, and others. Each type of dementia has its own distinct characteristics and underlying causes.

Although there is currently no cure for most types of dementia, there are treatments and interventions available that can help manage symptoms and improve quality of life for individuals with dementia. Early diagnosis and intervention are crucial for managing the condition and providing appropriate support and care. Treatment for dementia is based on the underlying cause, which is why diagnosis is very important.

DEPRESSION

Depression is a complex mental health condition characterized by persistent feelings of sadness, emptiness, or hopelessness, along with a loss of interest or pleasure in activities that were once enjoyable. It can impact various aspects of a person's life, including their thoughts, emotions, behaviors, and physical health. Other common symptoms may include changes in appetite or weight, sleep disturbances, fatigue, difficulty concentrating, feelings of worthlessness or guilt, and even thoughts of self-harm or suicide. Depression can range from mild to severe and can be triggered by a combination of genetic, biological, environmental, and psychological factors. It's important for individuals experiencing symptoms of depression to seek support from mental health professionals, as effective treatments, including therapy, medication, and lifestyle changes, can help manage and alleviate symptoms.

DIABETES (TYPE 2)

Type 2 diabetes is a metabolic disorder characterized by high blood sugar levels resulting from either insulin resistance or insufficient insulin production by the pancreas. Insulin, a hormone produced by the pancreas, helps regulate glucose uptake into cells for energy or storage. In insulin resistance, cells fail to respond effectively to insulin, causing glucose to accumulate in the bloodstream. Over time, the pancreas may lose its ability to produce enough insulin to compensate for this resistance, exacerbating high blood sugar levels.

Various factors contribute to the development of type 2 diabetes, including genetics, obesity, sedentary lifestyle, aging, and certain ethnicities. Excess body weight, especially around the abdomen, is a significant risk factor as it promotes insulin resistance. Physical inactivity further exacerbates insulin resistance and weight gain.

Diabetes must be carefully managed, because if not, there can be complications such as cardiovascular disease, neuropathy (nerve damage), nephropathy (kidney damage), retinopathy (eye damage), and increased susceptibility to infections. Management of type 2 diabetes involves lifestyle modifications such as adopting a healthy diet, regular exercise, weight management, and monitoring blood sugar levels. Medications, including oral antidiabetic drugs and insulin injections, may be prescribed to help control blood sugar levels when lifestyle changes alone are insufficient. Early diagnosis and proactive management are crucial for preventing or delaying complications associated with type 2 diabetes.

ERECTILE DYSFUNCTION

Erectile dysfunction (ED), also known as impotence, is a condition characterized by the consistent inability to achieve or maintain an erection sufficient for satisfactory sexual performance. It can affect men of all ages, but it becomes more common as men get older. ED can have various underlying causes, including physical factors such as cardiovascular disease, diabetes, hormonal imbalances, neurological disorders, and anatomical issues affecting the blood flow to the penis. Additionally, psychological factors like stress, anxiety, depression, and relationship problems can contribute to ED. Lifestyle factors such as smoking, excessive alcohol consumption, obesity, and lack of exercise can also increase the risk of developing ED.

Diagnosis of ED typically involves a physical examination, medical history review, and sometimes specialized tests such as blood tests, urine tests, or imaging studies. Treatment options range from oral medications like sildenafil (Viagra), tadalafil (Cialis), and vardenafil

(Levitra), to injections, vacuum devices, penile implants, hormone therapy, psychotherapy, and lifestyle modifications. The choice of treatment depends on the underlying cause of ED and individual preferences. Seeking medical advice is crucial for proper diagnosis and management of erectile dysfunction.

HEART DISEASE

Heart disease refers to a range of conditions that affect the heart. It's often used interchangeably with cardiovascular disease, which generally refers to conditions that involve narrowed or blocked blood vessels that can lead to a heart attack, chest pain (angina), or stroke.

Unfortunately, there are many types of heart disease; some of the most common are below.

Arrhythmias: These are irregular heartbeats, which can cause the heart to beat too quickly, too slowly, or irregularly.

Cardiomyopathy: This refers to diseases of the heart muscle, which can lead to heart failure.

Congenital heart defects: These are structural problems with the heart that are present at birth.

Coronary artery disease (CAD): This is the most common type of heart disease and is caused by the buildup of plaque in the coronary arteries, which supply blood to the heart muscle. This buildup can lead to angina, heart attack, or heart failure.

Heart failure: Also known as congestive heart failure, this occurs when the heart muscle is weakened and can't pump blood effectively.

Valvular disease: These can include stenosis (narrowing) or regurgitation (leakage) of the heart valves, which can affect blood flow through the heart.

There are many risk factors for heart disease, including high blood pressure, high cholesterol, smoking, diabetes, obesity, a sedentary lifestyle, and a family history of heart disease. Lifestyle changes are crucial in preventing and managing heart disease. Eating a healthy diet, exercising regularly, quitting smoking, and managing stress are just a few of these changes that can reverse heart disease or reduce the severity of the symptoms.

HIGH CHOLESTEROL

Cholesterol is a fatty substance that your body needs to function properly. However, when levels of cholesterol in the blood become too high, it can lead to health problems. High cholesterol, also known as hypercholesterolemia, refers to an excess of cholesterol in the bloodstream.

Cholesterol can be divided into two main types: low-density lipoprotein (LDL) and high-density lipoprotein (HDL). LDL cholesterol is often referred to as "bad" cholesterol because it can build up on the walls of arteries, forming plaque and narrowing the arteries (atherosclerosis), and an increased risk of heart disease and stroke. Conversely, HDL cholesterol is often called "good" cholesterol because it helps remove LDL cholesterol from the arteries.

High cholesterol typically does not cause symptoms, which is why it's important to have your cholesterol levels checked regularly through a blood test. Lifestyle factors such as diet, physical activity, and weight can influence cholesterol levels. In some cases, genetic factors can also play a role. Treatment often involves lifestyle changes such as adopting a healthy diet low in saturated and trans fats, increasing physical activity, quitting smoking, and maintaining a healthy weight. In some cases, medication may also be prescribed to help lower cholesterol levels, particularly if lifestyle changes alone are not sufficient.

HYPERTENSION
(HIGH BLOOD PRESSURE)

Hypertension, commonly known as high blood pressure, is a medical condition characterized by elevated pressure exerted by the blood against the walls of the arteries. Blood pressure is typically measured in millimeters of mercury (mmHg) and is expressed as two numbers: systolic pressure (the pressure in the arteries when the heart beats) over diastolic pressure (the pressure in the arteries when the heart rests between beats).

Normal blood pressure is typically considered to be around 120/80 mmHg. Hypertension is diagnosed when blood pressure consistently measures at 130/80 mmHg or higher. It's an important health concern because it can strain the heart, damage blood vessels, and increase the risk of serious health problems such as heart disease, stroke, and kidney disease.

Hypertension can often be managed through lifestyle changes such as maintaining a healthy diet, regular exercise, managing stress, limiting alcohol intake, and quitting smoking. In some cases, medication may also be necessary to control blood pressure levels. Regular monitoring and management of blood pressure are crucial in preventing complications associated with hypertension.

INFERTILITY

Infertility refers to the inability to conceive after a year of regular, unprotected sexual intercourse, or the inability to carry a pregnancy to term. It can affect both men and women and can be caused by various factors including but not limited to hormonal imbalances, reproductive system disorders, age, lifestyle factors, environmental factors, genetic factors, and certain medical conditions or treatments.

Infertility can be classified into primary infertility, which refers to couples who have never been able to conceive, and secondary infertility, which refers to couples who have conceived at least once but are unable to conceive again. Infertility can have significant emotional, psychological, and social impacts on individuals and couples, and it often requires medical intervention or assisted reproductive technologies to achieve pregnancy.

IRON DEFICIENCY

Iron deficiency is a condition characterized by insufficient levels of iron in the body. Iron is an essential mineral required for the production of hemoglobin, a protein in red blood cells that helps transport oxygen from the lungs to the rest of the body. When iron levels are low, the body's ability to produce an adequate amount of hemoglobin is compromised, leading to a condition known as iron deficiency anemia.

Iron deficiency can occur due to various factors, including inadequate dietary intake of iron, poor absorption of iron from the diet (often as a result of gastrointestinal disorders or surgeries), increased iron requirements (such as during pregnancy or periods of rapid growth), or chronic blood loss (e.g., through menstruation, gastrointestinal bleeding, or other medical conditions).

When the body is deficient of iron, many problems can develop, including fatigue, weakness, pale skin, shortness of breath, dizziness, headache, cold hands and feet, brittle nails, and unusual cravings for nonfood items (a condition called pica). In more severe cases, iron deficiency anemia can lead to complications such as heart problems and developmental delays in children.

Diagnosis of iron deficiency usually involves blood tests to measure levels of hemoglobin, serum iron, ferritin (a protein that stores iron), and other markers of iron status. In most cases, this condition is very treatable and typically involves iron supplementation, either through oral iron supplements or, in more severe cases or when oral supplements are not effective, through intravenous iron therapy. Identifying and addressing the underlying cause of iron deficiency is also important to prevent recurrence.

MUSCLE LOSS

Sarcopenia is a type of muscle atrophy associated with aging. It is a natural process characterized by a gradual loss of muscle mass, strength, and function that occurs with advancing age. Muscle atrophy associated with aging can have significant consequences, including decreased mobility, loss of balance, increased risk of falls and fractures, reduced quality of life, and loss of independence. However, regular physical activity, especially resistance training and aerobic exercise, along with a balanced diet rich in protein and nutrients, can help mitigate muscle loss and maintain strength and function as people age. Several factors contribute to muscle loss:

Chronic diseases: Conditions such as diabetes, heart disease, and arthritis, which become more prevalent with age, can also contribute to muscle atrophy due to inflammation, hormonal changes, or reduced physical activity.

Decreased protein synthesis: Aging is associated with a reduced ability of the body to synthesize proteins, which are essential for maintaining muscle mass.

Hormonal changes: Changes in hormone levels, such as decreased production of growth hormone, testosterone, and estrogen, can contribute to muscle loss and reduced muscle repair and regeneration.

Inflammation: Chronic low-grade inflammation, known as inflammageing, is common in older adults and can contribute to muscle wasting as well as frailty, cardiovascular disease, and death.

Mitochondrial dysfunction: Mitochondria, the energy-producing units of cells, may become less efficient with age, leading to decreased energy supply to muscles during exercise and daily activities.

Neurological changes: Age-related changes in the nervous system can affect the signals sent to muscles, leading to decreased muscle activation and strength.

Poor nutrition: Inadequate intake of protein and other essential nutrients can impair muscle maintenance and repair.

Reduced physical activity: As people age, they often become less physically active, leading to muscle disuse and atrophy. Sedentary lifestyles accelerate muscle loss.

OBESITY

Obesity is not an aesthetic judgment of someone's fatness, rather it's a medical condition characterized by an excessive accumulation of body fat, to the point where it may have a negative impact on health. It is typically measured using the Body Mass Index (BMI), which is calculated by dividing a person's weight in kilograms by the square of their height in meters (see this calculation in chapter 9). A BMI of 30 or higher is generally considered indicative of obesity.

Obesity can result from various factors, including genetics, lifestyle choices, dietary habits, physical activity levels, socioeconomic status, and environmental influences. It is associated with an increased risk of developing numerous health problems, such as type

2 diabetes, heart disease, stroke, certain cancers, osteoarthritis, and sleep apnea, among others.

Management and treatment of obesity typically involve a combination of dietary changes, increased physical activity, behavioral modifications, and sometimes medications or surgical interventions, depending on the severity of the condition and individual circumstances. Preventive measures such as adopting a healthy lifestyle, including balanced diet and regular exercise, are crucial in addressing and preventing obesity.

Dr. Ian's Tips

SPICE YOUR LIFE

Some of the greatest health promoters reside in those little jars and bottles in your pantry—herbs and spices. Derived from plants, these nutrition powerhouses can do more than make a bland piece of chicken or fish more appealing to your demanding taste buds. They carry their own dose of healthiness. Cinnamon has been shown to have potent antioxidant activity and anti-inflammatory effects, and helps lower cholesterol levels in the blood. Researchers believe that sage helps improve brain function and memory. Turmeric, the spice known to give curry its yellow coloring, contains a compound called curcumin that not only fights damage caused by oxidation but boosts the body's own antioxidant enzymes. There are all kinds of spices and herbs that are just an arm's length away that are ready to please your palate and boost your quest for overall good health.

OSTEOPOROSIS

Osteoporosis is a medical condition characterized by weakening of bones, leading to an increased risk of fractures. It occurs when the body loses too much bone, makes too little bone, or both. Bones that are not mineralized properly are less dense, making them brittle and fragile. Osteoporosis can affect any bone in the body, but fractures most commonly occur in the hip, spine, and wrist.

Risk factors for osteoporosis include aging, genetics, hormonal changes (such as menopause in women), certain medications, life-style factors (such as lack of exercise, excessive alcohol consumption, and smoking), and certain medical conditions (such as rheumatoid arthritis and conditions affecting hormone levels).

Prevention and management of osteoporosis involve lifestyle changes such as regular weight-bearing exercise, adequate intake of calcium and vitamin D, quitting smoking, limiting alcohol consump-tion, and medications prescribed by healthcare professionals to help strengthen bones and reduce fracture risk. Early detection through bone density testing can also aid in preventing complications associ-ated with osteoporosis.

OVERACTIVE BLADDER

Overactive bladder (OAB) is a urological condition characterized by a combination of urinary urgency, frequency, and sometimes urge in-continence, which is the involuntary leakage of urine. People with OAB often experience a sudden and intense urge to urinate, which may be difficult to control and can occur even when the bladder is not full. This urge may lead to frequent trips to the bathroom, disrupt-ing daily activities and sleep patterns. OAB can result from various underlying causes, including nerve damage, bladder inflammation, hormonal changes, or muscle dysfunction. Treatment strategies typ-ically involve a combination of lifestyle modifications (such as blad-der training, dietary changes, and fluid management), medications (such as anticholinergics or beta-3 agonists), pelvic floor exercises, and in some cases, minimally invasive procedures or surgery. OAB can significantly impact quality of life, but with appropriate manage-ment, symptoms can often be effectively controlled or improved.

PARKINSON'S DISEASE

Parkinson's disease is a neurodegenerative disorder that primarily affects movement. It develops gradually, often starting with minor tremors and stiffness before progressing to more severe symptoms. The condition occurs when certain nerve cells (neurons) in the brain that produce dopamine, a neurotransmitter responsible for transmitting signals that control movement, become impaired or die.

The exact cause of Parkinson's disease is still not fully understood, but both genetic and environmental factors are believed to play a role. Common symptoms of Parkinson's disease include tremors, stiffness or rigidity in the limbs, extreme slowness of movement and reflexes (bradykinesia), and impaired balance and coordination. As the disease progresses, individuals may also experience nonmotor symptoms such as cognitive changes, depression, sleep disturbances, and autonomic dysfunction.

While there is currently no cure for Parkinson's disease, treatments are available to help manage symptoms and improve quality of life. These treatments may include medications that increase dopamine levels in the brain, deep brain stimulation (DBS) surgery, physical therapy, and lifestyle modifications. Ongoing research continues to explore potential causes, risk factors, and treatments for Parkinson's disease.

PREDIABETES

Prediabetes is a condition characterized by higher-than-normal blood sugar levels, but not high enough to be classified as type 2 diabetes. It's considered a warning sign that you may be at risk for developing type 2 diabetes if steps are not taken to improve lifestyle habits. People with prediabetes have blood sugar levels that are higher than normal, but not yet high enough to be diagnosed as diabetes.

Prediabetes often doesn't have any symptoms, so many people may have it without knowing. However, it can be detected through blood tests that measure blood glucose levels. Lifestyle changes such as adopting a healthy diet, increasing physical activity, and losing weight can often prevent or delay the onset of type 2 diabetes in people with prediabetes. Regular monitoring and management of blood sugar levels are essential for individuals with prediabetes to prevent or delay the progression to type 2 diabetes.

RHEUMATOID ARTHRITIS

Rheumatoid arthritis (RA) is an autoimmune disorder that primarily affects the joints. In autoimmune diseases, the body's immune system mistakenly attacks its own tissues. In the case of rheumatoid arthritis, this immune response targets the synovium, which is the lining of the membranes that surround the joints. This chronic inflammatory disorder can lead to painful swelling, stiffness, and eventually joint damage and deformity. RA commonly affects joints in the hands, wrists, knees, and feet, but it can also involve other organs and systems of the body.

The exact cause of rheumatoid arthritis is not fully understood, but it is believed to involve a combination of genetic, environmental, and hormonal factors. There is no cure for RA, but various treatments, including medications, physical therapy, and lifestyle changes, can help manage symptoms, slow the progression of the disease, and improve the quality of life for those affected. Early diagnosis and treatment are crucial in minimizing joint damage and disability associated with RA.

SLEEP DISORDERS

Sleep disorders are a group of conditions that affect the ability to get quality sleep on a regular basis. They can disrupt normal sleep patterns and cause difficulties in falling asleep, staying asleep, or achieving restful sleep. Sleep disorders can be caused by various factors including medical conditions, mental health disorders, lifestyle choices, or environmental factors. There are numerous sleep disorders, but some of the more common ones are below:

Circadian rhythm disorders: Disruptions to the body's internal clock, leading to difficulties in falling asleep and waking up at desired times. Examples include delayed sleep phase disorder, advanced sleep phase disorder, and shift work sleep disorder.

Insomnia: Characterized by difficulty falling asleep, staying asleep, or waking up too early and not being able to fall back asleep. It can be acute (short-term) or chronic (long-term).

Narcolepsy: A neurological disorder characterized by excessive daytime sleepiness and sudden attacks of sleep, as well as other symptoms such as cataplexy (sudden loss of muscle tone triggered by strong emotions) and vivid hallucinations when falling asleep or waking up.

Parasomnias: Abnormal behaviors or movements during sleep, including sleepwalking, sleep talking, nightmares, night terrors, and REM sleep behavior disorder (acting out dreams during REM sleep).

Restless legs syndrome (RLS): An uncontrollable urge to move the legs, often accompanied by uncomfortable sensations in the legs. Symptoms typically worsen in the evening and at night, leading to difficulty falling asleep.

Sleep apnea: A condition where breathing repeatedly stops and starts during sleep. There are two main types: obstructive sleep apnea, caused by a blockage of the airway, and central sleep apnea, caused by a problem with the brain's signaling to the muscles that control breathing.

Sleep-related movement disorders: Conditions characterized by abnormal movements or behaviors during sleep, such as periodic limb movement disorder (PLMD) and bruxism (teeth grinding).

Proper diagnosis and treatment by a healthcare professional are important for managing sleep disorders effectively.

TESTICULAR CANCER

Testicular cancer is a type of cancer that develops in the testicles, which are part of the male reproductive system. Testicular cancer usually begins in the germ cells, which are the cells in the testicles that produce sperm. It is one of the less common types of cancer, but it is also one of the most treatable, especially when detected early.

There are two main types of testicular cancer:

Seminoma: This type of testicular cancer tends to grow and spread more slowly than nonseminoma. It is often highly treatable, even when it has spread beyond the testicle.

Nonseminoma: This type of testicular cancer tends to grow and spread more quickly than seminoma. Nonseminoma tumors are made up of different cell types, including embryonal carcinoma, yolk sac carcinoma, choriocarcinoma, and teratoma. Treatment and prognosis can vary depending on the specific types of cells involved.

Testicular cancer typically presents as a painless lump or swelling in one of the testicles. Other symptoms can include a feeling of heaviness in the scrotum, enlargement or tenderness of the breasts, back pain, and fluid collection in the scrotum. However, many men with testicular cancer may not experience any symptoms at all.

Treatment for testicular cancer has been well tested and tends to be quite effective when the cancer is localized and hasn't spread. Treatment usually involves surgery to remove the affected testicle, a procedure called orchiectomy. Additional treatments such as chemotherapy, radiation therapy, or lymph node surgery may be recommended depending on the type and stage of the cancer.

Regular testicular self-exams and routine medical checkups are important for early detection and treatment of testicular cancer.

The Inspiration

Jack, a 45-year-old sales manager, started noticing some unusual symptoms over a few months. He experienced frequent thirst, increased hunger despite maintaining his usual diet, and occasional blurry vision. Concerned about his health, he decided to schedule an appointment with his primary care physician.

During his visit, Jack's physician conducted a thorough examination and ordered several tests, including a fasting blood glucose test and an HbA1c test to assess his blood sugar levels over the past few months. The results revealed that Jack had elevated blood glucose levels, indicating prediabetes.

The Plan

Jack's physician immediately discussed the implications of his test results and the importance of managing his blood sugar levels to prevent the development of type 2 diabetes. Together, they formulated a comprehensive plan:

Dietary modifications: Jack consulted with a nutritionist to create a personalized meal plan focused on whole foods, complex carbohydrates, lean proteins, and healthy fats. He learned to monitor portion sizes and limit his intake of sugary and processed foods.

Regular exercise: Jack committed to increasing his physical activity by incorporating regular exercise into his daily routine. He started by walking for 30 minutes each day, and gradually progressed to more intensive workouts, including strength training and more intensive cardiovascular exercises.

Medication management: While Jack's physician initially recommended lifestyle changes as the primary approach, they also discussed the option of medication to help regulate his blood sugar levels if necessary. However, Jack responded well to lifestyle modifications and did not require medication at this stage.

Monitoring and follow-up: Jack's physician scheduled regular follow-up appointments to monitor his progress, adjust his treatment plan as needed, and provide ongoing support and encouragement.

The Change

Thanks to his proactive approach to his health and the timely intervention of his healthcare team, Jack successfully managed his prediabetes. By adhering to his diet and exercise regimen, he was able to stabilize his blood sugar levels and prevent the progression to type 2 diabetes. Regular monitoring and follow-up appointments ensured that

Jack remained vigilant about his health and continued to make positive lifestyle choices. Jack's case highlights the importance of paying attention to warning signs and seeking medical advice promptly. Through early detection and comprehensive management strategies, individuals like Jack can take control of their health and reduce their risk of developing serious chronic conditions such as type 2 diabetes.

3

YOUR TOP 10 POWER NUTRIENTS

Eating a healthy, well-balanced diet is something that should, of course, be done at every age. However, each decade of our life presents different challenges that we must face as we age and as our bodies evolve. The health concerns that you need to be aware of in your 30s might not be as important as the ones you might face in your 50s or 70s. While it's always good to get a full complement of vitamins, minerals, and other nutrients, there are certain ages where particular nutrients are higher up on the priority list because your body's needs change, as do the health conditions that are most likely to develop.

What are the nutrients you need to focus on and what are the best food sources that contain those nutrients? This chapter breaks it all down for you so that you can immediately assess what you need, what you've been lacking, and what you can do to fill the gap so that your nutrition plan gives you the best chance at fighting off disease, staying healthy longer, and avoiding the unnecessary pain and suffering that comes with so many chronic ailments. Just because a nutrient or food source is not listed under your current decade, it doesn't mean that it's not helpful in achieving good, long-lasting health. In fact, the best way to use this chapter is to look at the other decades, learn about nutrients that are not listed in your decade, and add them

NUTRIENTS

Antioxidants	Potassium
Calcium	Probiotics
Carbs	Protein
Fiber	Vitamin B_6
Iron	Vitamin B_9
Magnesium	Vitamin B_{12}
Monounsaturated fats	Vitamin C
Omega-3s	Vitamin D

30s	40s	50s	60s+
Calcium	Antioxidants	Antioxidants	Calcium
Carbs	Calcium	Calcium	Fiber
Fiber	Fiber	Fiber	Magnesium
Iron	Iron	Monounsaturated fats	Omega-3s
Magnesium	Magnesium	Omega-3s	Potassium
Omega-3s	Monounsaturated fats	Protein	Protein
Protein	Omega-3s	Vitamin B_9	Vitamin B_6
Probiotics	Potassium	Vitamin B_{12}	Vitamin B_9
Vitamin B_6	Vitamin B_{12}	Vitamin C	Vitamin B_{12}
Vitamin B_9	Vitamin D	Vitamin D	Vitamin D

to your nutritional regimen. Remember, it's never too early to adopt healthy changes.

YOUR 30s

This is a pivotal decade that really sets the stage for the rest of your life. It's easy to coast during these years, because you're feeling and looking good and you haven't had any serious illnesses. You're not thinking about heart disease or osteoporosis, because those are illnesses that most often afflict people much older than you. You're not thinking about nerve problems or dementia, because they are believed to be illnesses of the elderly, and thankfully you are many decades away from joining that group. While this type of thinking is common, it can also be costly. A lot of illnesses that we experience in middle age and older are typically set up by the way we live our life in our 30s and 40s. By focusing on a few important nutrients and foods now, you can receive large returns on your nutritional investment for years to come.

YOUR 40s

This is the decade where we really start to see signs of aging, both externally and internally. For most people, this will be the halfway point of their life. Not only is the timeline going to start shortening, but all the food, exercise (or lack of), environments we've lived in, stress, and self-care choices will start to take hold and manifest. This is the decade where you might get your first glimpse or consideration of your mortality. You might receive your first serious medical diagnosis or, for the first time, your physician reveals there are some test results that are concerning and need to be monitored. You might be under a lot of pressure from things such as family, job, and finances. You might also experience the startling realization that you're no longer the youngest person in the room, and that many life situations you had always felt were so far down the road are actually here. What you eat and how you treat yourself in this decade are critical in setting up the next 30 to 40 years of your life. If you haven't been focused and diligent about how you nourish and treat your body, now is the time you absolutely must get serious.

YOUR 50s

For many, this is *the* defining decade where you can't take your health for granted, and if you do, you do so at your own peril. This is a pivotal decade as it relates to health concerns. Issues with blood sugar regulation (prediabetes and diabetes), heart disease, high blood pressure, and joint ailments are just some of the many challenges you might face. The good news is that for most people it's not too late to make some dietary and physical changes that can get your health train back on the right track. Your metabolism is going to slow down and your ability to process certain foods can also hit a speed bump. That 8-ounce ribeye you are accustomed to eating doesn't work its way through your digestive system as easily as it did the previous couple of decades. Jumping out of bed and rushing into your daily routine might not be as painless as it was before, with your joints and soft tissues creaking and clicking and reminding you they need more time to warm up. You really need to watch what's on your plate and get up from your bed or sofa and start moving. What you eat always matters regardless of what decade of life you're in, but this is the decade where it really counts. A few changes in your nutritional and exercise regimens can go a long way in keeping you out of your doctor's office and enjoying your life uninterrupted by medical situations that can cost you not only a lot of time but also a lot of money.

YOUR 60s

This has long been considered the golden decade of our life, where we have lived most of our years and the pressures and concerns that dominated the previous decades have shifted dramatically. This is the decade where many people get serious about happiness and settle on a priority list that has little to do with material wealth and acquisitions and more to do with family, friends, and legacy. If you are fortunate to live this long, you have certainly been a witness to the highs and lows of life and all the curveballs that it pitches when least expected. These are years where you're not looking to start or establish a career, rather you're looking to wind things down and transition to a life filled with less career obligations and more leisure activities. The last 60 years have put a lot of wear and tear on your body and most likely you have the scars and medication bottles to show it. This, however, by no means indicates the end of your life is near or that your best years are behind you. In fact, some studies have found that more people in their 60s say they're "very happy" than those under the age of 35. You still have a lot of living to do and great memories still to be made; however, to take advantage of these opportunities, making your health a priority is pivotal. Taking care of your body and keeping it in the best shape possible means fueling it well and staying physically active. You're at an age where a little bit can truly go a long way.

NUTRIENTS AND FOOD SOURCES

Antioxidant

- apples
- artichokes
- beans
- beets
- blackberries
- blueberries
- broccoli
- carrots
- collard greens
- cranberries
- dark chocolate
- goji berries
- kale
- pecans
- potatoes
- prunes
- pumpkins
- raspberries
- red cabbage
- spinach
- squash
- strawberries

Calcium

- almonds
- breakfast cereals (fortified)
- broccoli
- cheese
- chia
- cottage cheese
- frozen yogurt
- kale
- milk (nonfat)
- mozzarella
- orange juice (fortified)
- salmon
- sardines
- soybeans
- soymilk
- spinach
- tofu
- turnip greens
- whole milk
- yogurt

Carbs

- almonds
- butter beans

- butternut squash
- carrots
- cashews
- chickpeas
- green lentils
- kidney beans
- parsnips
- pinto beans
- quinoa
- red lentils
- sweet potato
- walnuts
- yam

Fiber

- apples
- black beans
- bran
- chia seeds
- chickpeas
- flaxseeds
- guava
- popcorn
- peanuts
- raspberries
- seaweed
- squash
- soybeans (edamame)
- split peas
- sunflower seeds

Iron

Animal Based (Heme Iron)

- beef
- clams
- lamb chops
- oysters
- pork loin
- roasted chicken

- roasted turkey
- shrimp

Non-animal Based (Nonheme Iron)

- apricots
- beans (lima, navy, kidney)
- bran flakes
- cantaloupe
- fortified cereals, cream of wheat
- mustard greens
- nuts (walnuts, almonds, cashews)
- prunes
- raisins
- spinach
- tomato juice

Magnesium

- almonds
- baked potato with skin
- banana
- beef
- black beans
- broccoli
- brown rice
- cashews
- chia seeds
- chicken breast
- edamame
- fortified breakfast cereals
- kidney beans
- oatmeal
- peanut butter
- peanuts
- plain yogurt
- roasted pumpkin seeds
- salmon
- soymilk

- spinach
- whole-wheat bread

Monounsaturated Fats

- corn oil
- flaxseeds
- mackerel
- pumpkin seeds
- safflower oil
- salmon
- sardines
- sesame oil
- soybean oil
- sunflower oil

Omega-3s

Fish and Other Seafood

- herring
- mackerel
- salmon
- sardines
- tuna

Fortified Foods

- eggs
- juices
- milk
- soy beverages
- yogurt

Nuts and Seeds

- chia seeds
- flaxseeds
- hemp seeds
- walnuts

Plant Oils

- canola oil
- flaxseed oil
- soybean oil

Potassium

- avocado
- bananas
- beans (kidney, lima, pinto, soy)
- beet greens
- bran cereal
- broccoli
- cantaloupe
- cashews
- chicken
- coconut water
- cucumbers
- dairy and plant milks (soy, almond)
- dried fruits (raisins, apricots)
- fish (cod, halibut, trout, tuna, rockfish)
- lentils
- mushrooms
- nuts
- orange juice
- oranges
- peas
- potatoes (white and sweet)

Probiotics

- fermented dairy
- fermented soybeans
- fermented vegetables
- kefir
- kimchi
- kombucha
- miso
- pickles
- sauerkraut
- semi-hard cheeses (cheddar, gouda, Havarti, Gruyère
- tempeh
- yogurt

Protein

Animal Sources

- chicken (skinless)
- egg
- ham
- lamb
- lobster
- pork
- salmon
- scallops
- shrimp
- steak, turkey
- tuna

Non-animal Sources

- black beans
- black-eyed peas
- chickpeas
- edamame
- fava beans
- green peas
- kamut
- lentils
- lima beans
- pinto beans
- quinoa
- red kidney beans
- spinach
- wheat berries

Nuts and Seeds

- almonds
- chia seeds
- flaxseeds
- peanut butter
- peanuts
- pistachios
- pumpkin seeds
- soy nuts
- sunflower seeds

Dairy Products

- cottage cheese (1% fat)
- Greek yogurt
- mozzarella
- regular milk
- regular yogurt
- skim milk
- soy milk
- string cheese (nonfat)

Vitamin B$_6$

- bananas
- beef
- brown rice
- cantaloupe
- chicken
- chickpeas
- collard greens
- eggs
- fortified cereals
- green peas
- kale
- orange
- papaya
- salmon
- spinach
- sunflower seeds
- sweet potato
- tuna
- turkey

Vitamin B$_9$

- asparagus
- avocado
- banana
- beans

- black-eyed peas
- broccoli
- Brussels sprouts
- cantaloupe
- eggs
- fortified breakfast cereals
- green peas
- kidney beans
- liver
- milk
- mustard greens
- oranges
- papaya
- peanuts
- romaine lettuce
- spaghetti
- spinach
- turnip greens
- white rice
- whole grains

Vitamin B$_{12}$

- chicken
- dairy products (cheese, milk, yogurt)
- eggs
- enriched soy or rice milk
- fish/shellfish (clams, salmon, sardines, trout)
- fortified breakfast cereals
- fortified nutritional yeast
- liver
- red meat

Vitamin C

- bell peppers
- black currants
- cantaloupe
- cherries

- chile peppers
- citrus fruits (grapefruit, lemons, kiwi, oranges)
- cruciferous vegetables (broccoli, Brussels sprouts, cabbage, cauliflower)
- guava
- kale
- mustard spinach
- papaya
- strawberries
- sweet potatoes
- tomatoes
- white potatoes

Vitamin D

- avocado
- bananas
- beet greens
- beans (kidney, lima, pinto, soy)
- bran cereal
- broccoli
- cantaloupe
- cashews
- chicken
- coconut water
- cucumbers
- dried fruits (raisins, apricots)
- dairy and plant milks (soy, almond)
- fish (cod, halibut, trout, tuna, rockfish)
- lentils
- mushrooms
- nuts
- oranges
- orange juice
- peas
- potatoes (white and sweet)

ANTIOXIDANTS

Antioxidants are special substances that help protect our cells against the constantly menacing molecules called free radicals. When the body breaks down food or is exposed to radiation or tobacco smoke, these free radicals are produced by default. In essence, they are just a byproduct and not produced intentionally. Unfortunately, they are extremely dangerous in that they can damage cells by impairing certain molecules such as DNA, lipids, proteins, and carbohydrates. Scientists have shown that free radicals potentially play a role in several diseases including cancer, heart disease, cataract formation, and inflammatory disease. Antioxidants prevent the damage caused by free radicals by preventing their formation, facilitating their decomposition, and helping with their elimination.

There isn't just one type of antioxidant. Fortunately, there is a long list of them, which makes our job of finding the foods that contain them a lot easier. On the next page you'll find a table of foods that will help your body boost its defenses against disease.

CALCIUM

Calcium is the most abundant mineral in the body. We can get calcium in many ways, including foods, medicines, and dietary supplements. Calcium occurs naturally in some foods and can be added (fortified) to others. We most often talk about calcium with regard to bone health, because almost all calcium in the body (98 percent) is stored in the bones and we use this storage as a reservoir to maintain proper calcium levels in the body. Calcium is also important for strong, healthy teeth and plays a role in many important processes in the body including muscle contraction, regulating normal heart rhythms, nerve function, and blood clotting. Consuming enough calcium in our foods is important, because if we fall short, the body will

ANTIOXIDANTS AND FOOD SOURCES

Allium sulfur compounds	Leeks, onions, and garlic
Anthocyanins	Eggplant, grapes, and berries
Beta-carotene	Pumpkin, mangoes, apricots, carrots, spinach, and parsley
Catechins	Red wine and tea
Copper	Seafood, lean meat, milk, and nuts
Cryptoxanthins	Red capsicum, pumpkin, and mangoes
Flavonoids	Tea, green tea, citrus fruits, red wine, onions, and apples
Indoles	Cruciferous vegetables such as broccoli, cabbage, and cauliflower
Isoflavonoids	Soybeans, tofu, lentils, peas, and milk
Lignans	Sesame seeds, bran, whole grains, and vegetables
Lutein	Green leafy vegetables like spinach, and corn
Lycopene	Tomatoes, apricots, pink grapefruit, and watermelon
Manganese	Seafood, lean meat, milk, and nuts
Polyphenols	Herbs (basil, cinnamon, cumin, oregano, parsley, rosemary, sage, thyme, turmeric)
Selenium	Seafood, offal, lean meat, and whole grains
Vitamin A	Liver, sweet potatoes, carrots, milk, and egg yolks
Vitamin C	Oranges, blackcurrants, kiwifruit, mangoes, broccoli, spinach, capsicum, and strawberries
Vitamin E	Vegetable oils (such as wheat germ oil), avocados, nuts, seeds, and whole grains
Zinc	Lean meat, milk, nuts, and seafood

Source: Department of Health Victoria, Australia Better Health Channel

compensate by removing the calcium stored in our bones. This loss of bone calcium can be endured for a certain period, but if it's not replaced accordingly, this can lead to thinner and weaker bones and an array of problems including fractures. Vitamin D is calcium's partner as it is required for calcium to be absorbed in the gut so that adequate calcium levels in the blood can be maintained. Because these partners work together, a deficiency of vitamin D can also lead to a deficiency of calcium, and this, in turn, can lead to a cascade of unfortunate medical conditions.

RECOMMENDED DIETARY ALLOWANCES (RDA) FOR CALCIUM

AGE	FEMALE	PREGNANT	LACTATING	MALE
19–50 years	1000 milligrams	1000 milligrams	1000 milligrams	1000 milligrams
51–70 years	1200 milligrams			1000 milligrams
Greater than 70 years	1200 milligrams			1200 milligrams

Source: Institute of Medicine

CARBOHYDRATES (SLOW-BURNING)

Slow-burning, also called slow-release, carbohydrates are important because they provide a sustained, slower release of energy. Carbs are without question the body's primary source of energy. They are vital in our diets, because they deliver the crucial energy that keeps us going. When we eat carbs, the digestive system breaks them down into glucose, which then enters the bloodstream and is carried to the cells for energy. However, the rate at which the body breaks down carbs and releases this energy is different. Some carbs release their energy slowly, and some release it quickly. Each type of carb can be beneficial at different times for different reasons, but slow-burning carbs are highlighted here because they can maintain steady blood glucose levels, sustain energy levels, help with weight loss, lower cholesterol levels, and improve cardiovascular health.

FIBER

Fiber is a type of carbohydrate the body can't digest. As mentioned above, carbohydrates are broken down in the body into sugar molecules called glucose. Because fiber can't be broken down, it travels through the digestive tract relatively intact. It can help keep our blood sugar levels in check, lower cholesterol levels, maintain bowel health, and keep hunger at bay. There's also a belief that fiber can lengthen one's life through something called telomeres, protein structures that are part of our DNA. They are located at both ends of our chromosome strands and help protect our genes (DNA sequences) and fight off diseases. Telomeres naturally shorten as we age, but there are behaviors and environmental conditions that can expedite this shortening. They include poor diet, obesity, smoking, stress, and poor quality of sleep. Though the science is complicated and the research is still being defined, the prevailing belief is that longer telomeres means a longer life, and shorter telomeres mean a shorter life. According to a study published in the scientific journal *Nutrients*, it's believed that fiber can help lengthen telomeres.[1]

RECOMMENDED DIETARY ALLOWANCES (RDA) FOR FIBER

	50 YEARS OLD AND YOUNGER	51 YEARS OLD AND OLDER
Men	38 grams	30 grams
Women	25 grams	21 grams

Source: *Institute of Medicine*

IRON

Iron is an important mineral that's needed for optimal growth and development. It can be found naturally in our foods and in supplements. The two forms of dietary iron are heme and nonheme. Heme iron can mostly be found in foods like fish, meat, and poultry. It is better absorbed than the nonheme iron that is found mostly in plant-based foods. Iron is fundamental in aiding the body to make hemoglobin, the protein in red blood cells that carries oxygen from our lungs to all parts of the body. Iron is also crucial in helping to produce myoglobin, the protein that supplies our muscles with oxygen. Additionally, iron plays an important role in the creation of certain hormones, those critical chemical messengers in the body. Iron deficiency (low iron levels) affects approximately ten million Americans and about half of these have been diagnosed as having iron deficiency anemia. The good news is that it's relatively easy to increase and maintain iron levels for most people. The amount of iron we need each day depends on age, gender, and whether most of your diet is plant-based or animal-based. Vegetarians and vegans need almost double the intake of iron listed in the table on the next page, because the body doesn't absorb the nonheme iron found in plant foods as effectively as it absorbs the heme iron found in animal food products.

Dr. Ian's Tip

FORAGE FOR FATTY FISH

Fish has one of the best combinations of protein and healthy fat. The best type of fish is the fatty type, such as salmon, black cod, mackerel, herring, bluefin tuna, whitefish, and striped bass, which are loaded with the all-important omega-3 fatty acids as well as vitamins B_2, D, calcium, phosphorus, iron, zinc, magnesium, iodine, and potassium. Studies have shown that people who consume fish regularly have a lower risk of dementia, heart disease, and inflammatory bowel disease.

RECOMMENDED DIETARY ALLOWANCES (RDAS) FOR IRON

AGE	FEMALE	PREGNANCY	LACTATION	MALE
19–50 years	18 milligrams	27 milligrams	9 milligrams	8 milligrams
51+ years	8 milligrams			8 milligrams

Source: Institute of Medicine

MAGNESIUM

Magnesium is one of the body's most important minerals. It is naturally found in a variety of foods but is also available in supplements. About 60 percent of the body's magnesium is found in the bones, while the remaining inventory can be found in blood, muscles, and other soft tissue. Magnesium is a helper in the biochemical reactions that involve many processes, including muscle movements, bone health maintenance, proper nerve signaling, protein formation, and creation and repair of our genetic material (DNA and RNA).

RECOMMENDED DIETARY ALLOWANCE (RDA) FOR MAGNESIUM

AGE	FEMALE	PREGNANCY	LACTATION	MALE
19–30	310–320 milligrams	350 milligrams	310 milligrams	400 milligrams
31–50	350–360 milligrams	360 milligrams	320 milligrams	410 milligrams
51+	310–320 milligrams			420 milligrams

Source: Institute of Medicine

MONOUNSATURATED FATS

Most people tend to classify all fats as unhealthy, but the truth is that there are good fats and bad fats. Monounsaturated fats (MUFAs) are considered to be good fats because they help increase the good HDL (high density lipoprotein) cholesterol levels in our body and lower the bad LDL (low density lipoprotein) cholesterol levels that can lead to stroke and heart disease. MUFAs are one of two types of unsaturated fats, the other being polyunsaturated fats. Unsaturated fats get their name from their chemical structure. Oils that contain monounsaturated fats are physically liquid at room temperature but start to turn solid when chilled. Both monounsaturated and polyunsaturated fats are healthy fats, especially compared to the unhealthy saturated fats. The key is to simply remember: Unsaturated equals healthy and saturated equals unhealthy.

The difference between monounsaturated and polyunsaturated fats lies in their chemical structure. Without delving too deeply into the complicated science, the most important differences to know are that MUFAs are made by the body and are consumed in our foods, whereas polyunsaturated fats can't be made by the body and must come from food. Both types of unsaturated fats offer health benefits, and they contribute to the development and maintenance of the body's cells. Polyunsaturated fats also help lower LDL cholesterol levels, and they include omega-3 and omega-6 fats that are needed for brain function and cell growth and promote good heart health (omega-3) and potentially help control blood sugar (omega-6).

OMEGA-3S

These important fatty acids are abundant in our body as they are components of the membranes that surround each of the billions of cells that make us who we are. They provide us with energy and also have a role in the functioning of our blood vessels, heart, hormone-production glands (endocrine system), immune system, and lungs. They have been associated with many health benefits both short and long term. Some of the short-term benefits include reduced inflammation, improved sleep, better mood, and improved cognition. Some of the long-term benefits include improved eye health (reduced chances of macular degeneration), improved brain growth and development in infants, improved heart health, and improved bone and joint health. There are three main omega-3 fatty acids: alpha-linolenic acid (ALA), eicosapentaenoic acid (EPA), and docosahexaenoic acid (DHA). ALA is an essential fatty acid because our body can't make it. We must get it from food and beverages or supplements. Some of this ALA can be converted into EPA and DHA by our body but only in very small amounts, which is why we need to consume the proper portions of certain foods (flaxseed, canola oil, soybeans, walnuts, tofu) or supplements to boost their levels.

RECOMMENDED DIETARY ALLOWANCE (RDA) FOR ALA

	AMOUNT OF ALA
Men	1.6 grams
Women	1.1 grams
Pregnant	1.4 grams
Breastfeeding Women	1.3 grams

Source: Institute of Medicine
Note: Experts have not yet established recommended amounts of omega-3 fatty acids, except for ALA.

POTASSIUM

Potassium is a mineral that is critical for the body to function properly. It is one of many electrolytes, a group of minerals that have an electrical charge when they are dissolved in water or body fluids such as blood or urine. Potassium is found in all body tissue and is required for the normal functioning of cells. One of its main purposes is to help maintain normal levels of fluid inside our cells. This contrasts with another important electrolyte, sodium, which helps maintain normal fluid levels outside of the cells. Potassium is important for normal muscle contractions and helps maintain normal blood pressure. Our kidneys are important in regulating potassium levels as they help the body get rid of extra potassium through our urine. Too much potassium in the body (hyperkalemia) can be as dangerous as too little (hypokalemia), so it's important to be aware of your potassium levels should you experience certain symptoms.

ADEQUATE INTAKES (AI) FOR POTASSIUM

AGE	MEN	WOMEN	PREGNANCY	LACTATION
19–50 years	3,400 milligrams	2,600 milligrams	2,900 milligrams	2,800 milligrams
51+ years	3,400 milligrams	2,600 milligrams		

Source: National Academies of Sciences, Engineering, and Medicine

Symptoms of Potassium Excess and Deficiency

EXCESS

- Chest pain
- Irregular heart rate
- Heart palpitations
- Nausea
- Shortness of breath
- Weakness/fatigue

DEFICIENCY

- Constipation
- Fatigue
- Irregular heart rate (severe deficiency state)
- Muscle cramps or weakness
- Muscle paralysis (severe deficiency state)

PROBIOTICS

Our bodies are full of bacteria that, along with other microorganisms, are often thought to be detrimental to our health. However, not all of these "germs" are considered bad. In fact, some can be helpful and health-promoting. These "good" bacteria can be found in food sources such as yogurt and other fermented foods such as kimchi, sauerkraut, pickles, aged cheese, sour cream, miso, tempeh, and kombucha. Supplements also contain these helpful microorganisms, and we call these products probiotics. The most common of these probiotics contain bacteria typically belonging to the groups *Bifidobacterium* and *Lactobacillus,* but there are other bacteria and even some yeasts that are used as probiotics.

Researchers are still trying to detail how probiotics deliver their health benefits, but the generally accepted concept is that when levels of the "good" bacteria are lowered in the body (for example, when we take antibiotics that attack the bad bacteria but can also kill the good bacteria), probiotics can help to replace the good bacteria that have been lost. Scientists have also discovered that the gut (gastrointestinal tract) is an important center for our overall health. The gut is lined with both good and bad bacteria that exist in the proper balance for our bodies to function properly. When this balance is disrupted, we are vulnerable to developing illness. Probiotics are believed to help restore this important balance and deliver health-promoting benefits. Not all probiotics use the same type of microorganisms or in the same quantity. Just because a supplement claims to be a probiotic, it doesn't mean it's of high quality. Some of the characteristics you should consider before purchasing your probiotic include the amount of bacteria per dose, known as colony forming units (CFUs); which specific type of bacterial strains are used; whether the microorganisms being used have been studied for their effectiveness; and how the probiotic is supposed to be stored, as improper storage temperatures and conditions can reduce the lifespan and effectiveness of the bacteria, thus making it useless. Probiotics are generally considered safe; however, before starting any probiotic therapy, and particularly if you suffer from a medical condition, it would be prudent to check with your doctor to make sure it is safe for you.

Possible Medical Conditions Improved by Probiotics

- Diarrhea caused by antibiotics
- Infectious diarrhea
- Inflammatory bowel disease
- Irritable bowel disease
- Oral health
- Preventing/reducing allergy flares and limiting cold duration
- Skin conditions (like acne, atopic dermatitis, eczema, psoriasis, and rosacea)
- Urinary and vaginal health

Possible Probiotic Health Benefits

- Reduced stress and anxiety
- Boosted immune system
- Improved mood
- Improved nutrient absorption
- Lower cholesterol levels
- Improved illness recovery
- Reduced gas and bloating

PROTEIN

Proteins are made from amino acids that are linked together in a chain. Protein is found in every body part and tissue, including bone, hair, skin, and muscle. While our bodies can make protein, we must also consume adequate amounts of it so that our body can repair damaged cells and make new ones. Protein is one of the three macronutrients that our body needs in large supply. (Fats and carbohydrates are the other two.) Whether it's growing stronger muscles or replacing skin cells that die and slough away, proteins are part of the enzymes that facilitate thousands of chemical reactions that happen every second of our lives. Scientists have estimated that there are over 10,000 different proteins throughout our body, quietly carrying on critical life functions from smiling at a joke to lifting a bag of groceries from the trunk of a car.

How Much Protein Do You Need?

There are different recommendations for protein intake based on different variables, but the National Academy of Medicine recommends that most adults get at least 0.8 gram of protein for every kilogram of body weight. Another way of looking at it is that for every 20 pounds of body weight, you should consume just a little over 7 grams of protein. For example, someone who weighs 160 pounds should consume approximately 56 grams of protein each day.

Another way to make the calculation is by taking your weight in pounds and multiplying it by 0.36. So if you weigh 180 pounds, your daily protein requirement would be 0.36 x 180 = 64.8 grams.

VITAMIN B$_6$ (PYRIDOXINE)

This water-soluble vitamin is found naturally in many foods but is also added to foods and available in supplements. Vitamin B$_6$ is involved in immune function and fetal brain development during pregnancy as well as brain development during infancy. This vitamin is not only important during early development but throughout our life to maintain healthy immune and nervous systems. More than a hundred enzyme reactions that are involved in metabolism depend on the assistance of vitamin B_6. When taken in supplement form, the vitamin has shown some promise in treating pregnancy-induced nausea. According to the Harvard School of Public Health, maintaining sufficient levels of vitamin B_6 may be associated with lower risk of certain cancers. However, like any supplement, taking too much and having excessively high levels can be problematic, which is why it should only be taken under physician supervision in certain medical situations.

	AGE 19-50	AGE 51+
Female	1.3 milligrams	1.5 milligrams
Female Pregnant	1.9 milligrams	
Female Lactating	2.0 milligrams	
Male	1.3 milligrams	1.7 milligrams

VITAMIN B_9 (FOLATE)

Vitamin B_9 is found in many foods, but it also is found in supplements in a synthetic form called folic acid, which is better absorbed than the natural form in food sources. Folate has many functions and benefits in the body, including assisting in red blood cell formation, reducing the risk of birth defects of the brain and spine in newborns, and rapid cell growth and function. Folate also helps to form DNA and RNA at all stages of life and is involved in the building of proteins from amino acids. Not having enough vitamin B_9 in the blood can lead to a potentially health-compromising anemia in which your body produces abnormally large red blood cells that don't function properly. However, this condition can be easily avoided by consuming enough of it in either food or supplements or a combination of the two.

RECOMMENDED DIETARY ALLOWANCES (RDA) FOR FOLATE

	AGE 19+
Women	400 micrograms *DFE
Pregnant Women	600 micrograms DFE
Breastfeeding Women	500 micrograms DFE
Men	400 micrograms DFE

Source: National Institutes of Health

*DFE: dietary folate equivalents

VITAMIN B$_{12}$

Also known as cobalamin, vitamin B$_{12}$ has several important functions in the body, most notably helping with red blood cell formation, nerve function, cell metabolism, and the production of DNA. Since our body does not manufacture this vitamin, we must get it from our food. Vitamin B$_{12}$ binds to proteins that are found in animal-based foods. Once we eat these B$_{12}$-containing foods, the hydrochloric acid and enzymes in our stomach help free the B$_{12}$ from the protein. Once B$_{12}$ is free from the food protein, it now binds to a special protein produced by the stomach called intrinsic factor. This new intrinsic factor/vitamin B$_{12}$ unit travels down into the gastrointestinal tract until it reaches the small intestine, where the vitamin B$_{12}$ is then absorbed into blood vessels and can be used by the body.

Vitamin B$_{12}$ can be found in fortified foods (cereals, nutritional yeast, nondairy milk) and supplements. The vast majority of people who eat a balanced diet that includes some animal products are unlikely to develop a B$_{12}$ deficiency. However, those who don't eat animal products—vegans and some vegetarians—are at an increased risk of this deficiency because they are not getting adequate amounts of B$_{12}$ through their diet. Daily supplements can be helpful for those who don't or can't consume enough vitamin B$_{12}$.

RECOMMENDED DIETARY ALLOWANCES (RDA) FOR VITAMIN B$_{12}$

Men	2.4 micrograms
Women	2.4 micrograms
Pregnant Women	2.6 micrograms
Breastfeeding Women	2.8 micrograms

Source: National Institutes of Health

VITAMIN C

This water-soluble (dissolves in water) vitamin can also be recognized by the name ascorbic acid. Because it dissolves in water means that it is readily delivered to the body's tissues, but it also means that it can't be stored for future use and thus must be taken daily through food or supplements. Vitamin C has been known as the cold vitamin because it plays a role in controlling infections. It's a powerful antioxidant that can help with the healing of wounds and prevent damage caused by the destructive molecules called free radicals. It helps boost the body's immune system by stimulating the activity of white blood cells, the primary fighters that detect and fight infections or foreign substances that enter the body. We also need vitamin C to make collagen, the fibrous protein found in the connective tissue that weaves its way through the body like a spider web.

RECOMMENDED DIETARY ALLOWANCES (RDA) FOR VITAMIN C

Men 19+	90 milligrams
Women 19+	75 milligrams
Pregnant Women	85 milligrams
Breastfeeding Women	120 milligrams

Source: National Institutes of Health

Note: Individuals who smoke require 35 mg/day more vitamin C than nonsmokers.

VITAMIN D

Also known as calciferol, vitamin D is best known for its role in maintaining proper bone health. It helps the body absorb and retain calcium and phosphorus, two elements that we need for bone growth. Without sufficient levels of vitamin D in the body, bones can become thin or brittle and lead to diseases such as osteopenia and the more severe osteoporosis. According to the Harvard School of Public Health, research has shown that vitamin D can help reduce cancer cell growth, reduce inflammation, reduce the risk of heart attacks and strokes, reduce the severity of allergy flares, and help fight infections.

Vitamin D is a hormone our bodies can manufacture, and it's a nutrient contained in our food. There are not many food sources that contain naturally occurring vitamin D, rather several dairy products and breakfast cereals tend to be *fortified* with many nutrients, including vitamin D. When you see a food label that says it is fortified, that means the content of that micronutrient has been added or increased to improve the nutritional quality and provide a health benefit.

Vitamin D is also produced in the body when the ultraviolet rays from sunlight hit the skin, and this begins a series of chemical reactions that lead to vitamin D synthesis. To achieve optimal levels of vitamin D, we tend to rely on that found in foods as well as that made by the body due to sun exposure. People who are not eating a balanced diet or who have limited exposure to sunlight are at high risk of vitamin D deficiency and need to be vigilant about making sure their consumption/sunlight exposure is adequate. How much sunlight it considered adequate is not consistent for everyone, because it depends on where you are geographically, the season, and the time of day you get the sun exposure. The amount of time you need to be in the sun to produce adequate amounts of vitamin D can vary from just a few minutes in the summer in Miami to 23 minutes at noon if you're in Boston in the middle of winter. It's best to check with your healthcare provider or a dermatologist to assess how much sun exposure is considered healthy and adequate. However, sometimes just getting

RECOMMENDED DIETARY ALLOWANCES FOR VITAMIN D

19–70 years	15 micrograms (600 IU)
71 years and older	20 micrograms (800 IU)
Pregnant and breastfeeding women	15 micrograms (600 IU)

Sources: National Institutes of Health

more sun or eating fortified foods might not be enough to put your vitamin D levels within the normal range. A simple blood test can determine whether your levels are adequate or if they're deficient.

The Inspiration

Jackie, a 35-year-old marketing executive, led a busy life filled with long hours at work, frequent fast-food lunches, and minimal physical activity. Despite her demanding schedule, she noticed her health deteriorating. She often felt sluggish, struggled with excess weight, and her recent blood work revealed alarmingly high cholesterol levels.

The Plan

Motivated by a desire to reclaim her vitality and well-being, Jackie decided to make a radical change in her lifestyle. She embarked on a journey to prioritize nutritious food choices and incorporate regular exercise into her routine.

First, Jackie revamped her diet, replacing processed and high-fat foods with whole, nutrient-dense options. She started her day with a nutritious breakfast of oatmeal topped with fruits and nuts, instead of sugary pastries. For lunch, she swapped greasy fast food for homemade salads filled with colorful vegetables, lean proteins, and a variety of seeds. Her dinners consisted of grilled fish or chicken paired with steamed vegetables and whole grains.

In addition to her dietary changes, Jackie committed to exercising regularly. She incorporated brisk walks during her lunch breaks and scheduled gym sessions three times a week, focusing on a mix of cardiovascular exercises and strength training.

The Change

As Jackie adhered to her new lifestyle, remarkable transformations occurred. Within a few months, she began to notice significant changes in her health and well-being:

Weight loss: Jackie shed excess pounds steadily and healthily as a result of her improved eating habits and increased physical activity.

Lowered cholesterol levels: Regular consumption of nutritious foods, particularly those rich in fiber and healthy fats and other "power" nutrients, contributed to a notable reduction in Jackie's cholesterol levels, mitigating her risk of heart disease.

Increased energy: Jackie experienced a surge in energy levels throughout the day. By fueling her body with nutrient-rich foods and engaging in regular exercise, she found herself more alert, focused, and productive at work.

Improved mood and vitality: Gone were the days of feeling sluggish and lethargic. Jackie's newfound vitality and sense of well-being boosted her mood, confidence, and overall quality of life.

Through dedication, perseverance, and a commitment to prioritizing her health, Jackie successfully transformed her life. Her journey serves as a testament to the profound impact that wholesome nutrition and regular exercise can have on one's physical, mental, and emotional well-being. Jackie's story inspires others to take charge of their health and embark on their own transformative journeys toward a vibrant and fulfilling life.

4

YOUR 30-DAY MEAL PLAN

The following meal plans are just a guide for you to easily and abundantly incorporate your top 10 power nutrients into your diet, in order to help prevent or control some of those medical conditions most prevalent in your decade. These are not weight-loss plans; however, many people who follow them and do the suggested exercises will most likely lose weight. Feel free to switch the order of the days in the plan and substitute meals from one day to another. While quantities and portions are mentioned in the daily meals, you don't have to eat all the food that's listed, but rather eat until you're full but not stuffed.

You may have food allergies, taste preferences, medical conditions, access issues, or other factors that prevent you from strictly following the plan or eating the foods that are listed. Don't worry about it. Make the substitutions you need to and do your best to stick to the program. The main purpose of these plans is not to torment or bankrupt you, but rather to get you comfortable with eating those foods that will best serve you and give you the greatest opportunity to prevent disease and weight gain. You will be fueling your body in a way that will keep it highly functional and preserved so that aging will take the least amount of impact possible.

Have fun with the meal plans and feel free to create your own by being imaginative and exploring new foods and cuisines in your quest for maximal health. The 30-day meal plan below is just an example of what you can follow, but this is not just about 30 days; rather, this is how you'll be eating for most of your life. This is not meant to be a strict diet. Instead, it's a guideline to teach you how to choose and match the best foods with your power ingredients that will deliver great health benefits. Find your specific decade in this chapter and discover samples of some of the budget-conscience meal combinations that will appeal to not only your pallet but your health as well.

THE 30s

When it comes to nutrition, this decade is critical for constructing your body in a way that can be impactful for the rest of your life. Your body is still very flexible, which means it can change and adapt and transform with just a small amount of effort. Your bones and muscles need to be nourished with calcium and protein so that they are healthy and robust and can withstand the normal decline that will happen in the latter decades. Eating foods that are high in omega-3s are important for your brain and heart health, and the probiotics you consume can be instrumental in developing and maintaining a healthy gut. Look at this decade as building the strongest, healthiest, most nimble body that will be able to better withstand the challenges that aging will inevitably bring.

Below you will find some samples of different meals and snacks that incorporate the top 10 power nutrients for your decade. The quantity for each nutrient will depend on how much of the different foods you consume. There are numerous online nutrient calculators that will allow you to input the ingredients of the meals and give you an approximation of the nutrient quantities. Remember, these are only examples to give you an idea. There are infinite combinations of foods and recipes that you can choose from that will supply you with the various nutrients you need. It would not be possible to include them all in one book, let alone a single chapter.

BREAKFAST OPTIONS

- 2 scrambled eggs with spinach and feta cheese (protein, calcium, vitamin B_6)
- 1 slice whole-grain toast with your choice of topping (fiber, slow-burning carbs)
- 1½ cups oatmeal with chia seeds and sliced bananas (fiber, omega-3s, slow-burning carbs, magnesium)
- 2 scrambled eggs with smoked salmon and a whole-grain English muffin (protein, slow-burning carbs, omega-3s)
- 6 ounces scrambled tofu with spinach and 1 slice whole-grain toast with your choice of topping (protein, slow-burning carbs, fiber)
- 8-ounce Greek yogurt parfait with mixed berries and 2 tablespoons granola (protein, calcium, fiber)
- 2 small whole-grain waffles (6-inch diameter) with strawberries and a dollop of low-fat yogurt (fiber, vitamin B_9, slow-burning carbs, calcium)
- 10-ounce green smoothie with spinach, banana, and fortified almond milk (calcium, fiber, magnesium, vitamin B_6)
- 1½ cups oatmeal with flaxseeds, blueberries, and a dollop of Greek yogurt (fiber, omega-3s, protein, slow-burning carbs, calcium)
- 2 scrambled eggs with sautéed spinach, whole-grain toast, and a sprinkle of nutritional yeast (protein, vitamin B_6, slow-burning carbs, vitamin B_9)
- 2 small whole-grain pancakes (6-inch diameter) with almond butter and mixed berries (fiber, protein)
- 6 ounces scrambled tofu with sautéed kale and 1 slice whole-grain toast (protein, fiber, slow-burning carbs, calcium)
- 2 scrambled eggs with spinach and tomatoes (protein, vitamin B_6, fiber)
- 1½ cups oatmeal with sliced banana and almonds (fiber, protein, slow-burning carbs, monounsaturated fats)
- 2 scrambled eggs with spinach, whole-grain toast, and a side of

avocado (protein, fiber, slow-burning carbs, monounsaturated fats)

- 8-ounce Greek yogurt parfait with strawberries, honey, and granola (protein, calcium, slow-burning carbs, vitamin B_6)

LUNCH OPTIONS

- 6-ounce grilled boneless, skinless chicken breast with a side of quinoa (protein, vitamin B_6, fiber)
- 1 cup steamed broccoli (calcium, fiber, iron)
- mixed green salad with vinaigrette dressing made with flaxseed oil (omega-3s from flaxseed oil)
- 1½ cups lentil soup with a side salad (protein, iron, fiber)
- 6 ounces tofu stir-fry with broccoli, red bell peppers, and brown rice (antioxidants, fiber, protein, vitamin B6, vitamin B9)
- 2 cups quinoa salad with chickpeas, cucumbers, and tomatoes (protein, vitamin B_6)
- Grilled shrimp (4) salad with mixed greens, avocado, and a citrus vinaigrette (protein, omega-3s)
- Black bean and sweet potato burrito with a side of salsa (protein, fiber, vitamin B_9)
- Turkey and avocado wrap with a side of mixed greens (protein, fiber)
- 1½ cups lentil and vegetable soup with a side of mixed greens (protein, fiber, vitamin B_9)
- Turkey and avocado salad with mixed greens and a balsamic vinaigrette (protein, healthy fats, fiber)
- 1½ cups chickpea and vegetable curry with ½ cup brown rice (protein, fiber, vitamin B_9)
- Grilled shrimp (6) with ½ cup quinoa and roasted bell peppers (antioxidants, fiber, protein, vitamin B_6, vitamin B_9)
- 6 ounces grilled chicken breast salad with mixed greens and nuts (protein, vitamin B_6, magnesium, omega-3s)

- 2 cups lentil and vegetable stir-fry with ½ cup brown rice (protein, fiber, magnesium)
- Grilled shrimp (6) with quinoa and roasted bell peppers (antioxidants, fiber, protein, vitamin B_6, vitamin B_9)
- 6 ounces baked or grilled cod with ½ cup quinoa and 1 cup steamed Brussels sprouts (protein, omega-3s, fiber)
- 6 ounces grilled chicken with ½ cup brown rice and ½ cup steamed green beans (protein, slow-burning carbs)
- 6 ounces grilled salmon with ½ cup quinoa and ½ cup steamed broccoli (omega-3s, protein, calcium)
- 6 ounces grilled salmon with ½ cup quinoa and 4 medium roasted asparagus spears (omega-3s, protein, fiber)
- 6 ounces baked cod with ½ cup quinoa and 1 cup steamed Brussels sprouts (protein, omega-3s, fiber)
- 6 ounces grilled mackerel with ½ cup quinoa and ½ cup sautéed Swiss chard (protein, omega-3s, calcium)
- 1 cup beef stir-fry with ½ cup quinoa and ½ cup sautéed bok choy (protein, fiber, iron, calcium)
- Grilled shrimp (6) with quinoa and sautéed kale (protein, magnesium, fiber)
- 6 ounces grilled tofu with ½ cup broccoli and ½ cup brown rice

DINNER OPTIONS

- 6 ounces grilled or baked salmon, ½ cup mixed vegetables, 1 cup whole-grain pasta (omega-3s, fiber, slow-burning carbs, protein)
- 6-ounce grilled turkey breast with ½ cup quinoa and ½ cup steamed kale (protein, vitamin B_6, calcium)
- 6 ounces baked cod with ½ cup diced, roasted sweet potatoes and 4 medium asparagus spears (protein, vitamin B_6, calcium)
- 6 ounces grilled chicken with a side of ½ cup spinach, ½ cup brown rice, and ½ cup roasted beets (protein, iron, fiber)

- 2 cups beef stir-fry with ½ cup broccoli, ½ cup snap peas, and ½ cup brown rice (protein, iron)
- 6 ounces grilled mackerel with ½ cup quinoa and ½ cup sautéed Swiss chard (protein, omega-3s, calcium)
- 6-ounce grilled or baked boneless, skinless chicken breast with ½ cup quinoa and ½ cup steamed broccoli (protein, vitamin B_6, calcium)
- 2 cups quinoa salad with chickpeas, cucumbers, and tomatoes (protein, vitamin B_6)
- 6 ounces grilled salmon with quinoa and roasted asparagus (omega-3s, protein, fiber)
- 6 ounces baked cod with ½ cup quinoa and 1 cup steamed Brussels sprouts (protein, omega-3s, fiber)
- 6 ounces baked chicken with ½ cup brown rice and ½ cup steamed green beans (protein, slow-burning carbs)
- 6 ounces baked salmon with ½ cup steamed broccoli and ½ cup brown rice (omega-3s, protein, calcium, vitamin B_6, slow-burning carbs, magnesium)
- 6 ounces grilled tofu with ½ cup broccoli and ½ cup brown rice (calcium, fiber, iron, magnesium, protein)
- 2 cups beef stir-fry with ½ cup quinoa and ½ cup sautéed bok choy (protein, iron, calcium)
- Grilled shrimp (6) with ½ cup quinoa and ½ cup sautéed kale (protein, magnesium, fiber)
- 6 ounces grilled salmon with ½ cup quinoa and ½ cup steamed broccoli (omega-3s, protein, calcium)
- 6 ounces grilled mackerel with ½ cup quinoa and ½ cup sautéed Swiss chard (protein, omega-3s, calcium)

SNACK OPTIONS

- Greek yogurt (½ cup) with honey and chia seeds (protein, calcium, vitamin B_6, vitamin B_9, omega-3s, magnesium, fiber, whole grains)

- Cottage cheese (½ cup) with sliced almonds and berries (protein, calcium, vitamin B$_6$, vitamin B$_9$, omega-3s, magnesium, fiber, iron, whole grains)
- Edamame (1 cup) (protein, calcium, vitamin B$_6$, vitamin B$_9$, omega-3s, magnesium, fiber, iron, whole grains)
- Roasted chickpeas (1 cup) (protein, calcium, vitamin B$_6$, vitamin B$_9$, omega-3s, magnesium, fiber, iron, whole grains)
- Sardines (2) on whole-grain crackers (protein, calcium, vitamin B$_6$, vitamin B$_9$, omega-3s, magnesium, fiber, iron, whole grains)
- Hard-boiled eggs (1–2) with a side of spinach (protein, calcium, vitamin B$_6$, vitamin B$_9$, omega-3s, magnesium, fiber, iron, whole grains)
- Almond butter (1 tablespoon) on 1 slice of whole-grain toast with ½ banana, sliced (protein, calcium, vitamin B$_6$, vitamin B$_9$, omega-3s, magnesium, fiber, iron, whole grains)
- Hummus (3 tablespoons) with carrot and cucumber sticks (protein, calcium, vitamin B$_6$, vitamin B$_9$, omega-3s, magnesium, fiber, iron)
- Low-fat cheese (½ cup) and whole-grain pretzels (protein, calcium, vitamin B$_6$, vitamin B$_9$, omega-3s, magnesium, fiber, iron, whole grains)
- Quinoa salad with black beans, corn, and avocado (1 cup) (protein, calcium, vitamin B$_6$, vitamin B$_9$, omega-3s, magnesium, fiber, iron, whole grains)
- Trail mix with nuts, seeds, and dried fruit (¼ cup) (protein, calcium, vitamin B$_6$, vitamin B$_9$, omega-3s, magnesium, fiber, iron, whole grains)
- Spinach and feta–stuffed mushrooms (1 cup) (protein, calcium, vitamin B$_6$, vitamin B$_9$, omega-3s, magnesium, fiber, iron, whole grains)
- Tuna salad (½ cup with whole-grain crackers) (protein, calcium, vitamin B$_6$, vitamin B$_9$, omega-3s, magnesium, fiber, iron, whole grains)
- Pumpkin seeds (pepitas) and dark chocolate chips (½ cup to-

tal) (protein, calcium, vitamin B_6, vitamin B_9, omega-3s, magnesium, antioxidants, fiber, iron, whole grains)

- Baked sweet potato with almond butter (protein, calcium, vitamin B_6, vitamin B_9, omega-3s, magnesium, fiber, iron, whole grains)
- Whole-grain pita with guacamole and cherry tomatoes (protein, calcium, vitamin B_6, vitamin B_9, omega-3s, magnesium, fiber, iron, whole grains)
- Spinach and artichoke dip (3 tablespoons) with whole-grain tortilla chips (protein, calcium, vitamin B_6, vitamin B_9, omega-3s, magnesium, fiber, iron, whole grains)
- Lentil soup (1 cup) with a side of whole-grain bread (protein, calcium, vitamin B_6, vitamin B_9, omega-3s, magnesium, fiber, iron, whole grains)
- Muesli with nuts, seeds, and dried fruit (1 cup total): (protein, calcium, vitamin B_6, vitamin B_9, omega-3s, magnesium, fiber, iron, whole grains)
- Brown rice cakes (2) with cottage cheese and sliced peaches (protein, calcium, vitamin B_6, vitamin B_9, omega-3s, magnesium, fiber, iron, whole grains)

Now that you have some examples of the types of meals and snacks you can eat and the power nutrients they contain, you can mix and match them to create daily meal plans. Starting on the next page you will find menus with approximately 2,000 to 2,500 calories per day, but if you want to eat less, you can make adjustments to bring this calorie count lower. This is meant to be a stress-free, flexible plan that you will enjoy. You can make reasonable substitutions, such as swapping brown rice for quinoa and vice versa. You can mix days by taking meals or snacks from one day and substituting it in another day. For example, if you don't have the ingredients for dinner on day 2, but you have the ingredients for dinner on day 7, then you can have the day 7 dinner on day 2. The idea is to get as much of your top 10 power nutrients into your diet as possible and have fun while doing it.

30-DAY MEAL PLAN

DAY 1

Breakfast
- 2 scrambled eggs with spinach and feta cheese (protein, calcium, vitamin B_6)
- 1 slice whole-grain toast (fiber, slow-burning carbs)

Snack
- ½ cup Greek yogurt with berries (protein, calcium, vitamin B_9)
- 20 almonds (magnesium, healthy fats)

Lunch
- 6-ounce grilled boneless, skinless chicken breast with ½ cup quinoa (slow-burning carbs, protein, vitamin B_6, fiber)
- 1 cup steamed broccoli (calcium, fiber, iron)
- mixed green salad with vinaigrette dressing (omega-3s from flaxseed oil)

Snack
- 1 cup carrot and celery sticks with 2 tablespoons hummus (fiber, iron, protein, magnesium)

Dinner
- 6 ounces grilled or baked salmon (omega-3s, protein)
- 4 steamed asparagus spears (vitamin B_9, fiber)
- 1 cup whole-grain pasta (protein, fiber, slow-burning carbs)

DAY 2

Breakfast
- 1½ cups oatmeal with 1 tablespoon chia seeds and ¼ small banana, sliced (fiber, omega-3s, slow-burning carbs, magnesium)

Snack
- ½ cup cottage cheese with pineapple (calcium, iron, magnesium, protein, vitamin B_6)

Lunch
- 1½ cups lentil soup with a side salad (protein, iron, fiber)

Snack
- ½ cup mixed nuts (fiber, magnesium, monounsaturated fats, protein)

Dinner
- 6-ounce grilled turkey breast with ½ cup quinoa and ½ cup steamed kale (protein, vitamin B_6, calcium)

Snack
- 1 cup mixed berries of your choice with a dollop of Greek yogurt (vitamin B_9, protein)

DAY 3

Breakfast
- 2 small whole-grain pancakes (6-inch diameter) with 1 tablespoon almond butter and ½ cup blueberries (antioxidants, protein, fiber)

Snack
- 1 (3.5-ounce) tin of sardines on 4 small whole-grain crackers (omega-3s, calcium)

Lunch
- 6 ounces tofu stir-fry with broccoli, red bell peppers, and ½ cup brown rice (antioxidants, fiber, protein, vitamin B_6, vitamin B_9)

Snack
- 10-ounce green smoothie with spinach, banana, and fortified almond milk (calcium, fiber, magnesium, protein, vitamin B_9)

Dinner
- 6 ounces baked cod with ½ cup diced roasted sweet potatoes and 4 medium asparagus spears (protein, vitamin B_6, calcium)

Snack
- 2 ounces low-fat cheese with whole-grain crackers (calcium, fiber)

DAY 4

Breakfast
- 2 scrambled eggs with 3 ounces smoked salmon and 1 whole-grain English muffin (protein, fiber, slow-burning carbs, omega-3s)

Snack
- 10-ounce smoothie with kale, banana, chia seeds, and fortified almond milk (calcium, fiber, magnesium, protein)

Lunch
- 2 cups quinoa salad with chickpeas, cucumbers, and tomatoes (protein, fiber, slow-burning carbs, vitamin B$_6$)

Snack
- ¼ cup walnuts (omega-3s, magnesium)

Dinner
- 6 ounces grilled chicken with a side of ½ cup spinach, ½ cup brown rice, and ½ cup roasted beets (protein, iron, fiber)

Snack
- 6 ounces low-fat yogurt with honey (calcium, vitamin B$_9$)

DAY 5

Breakfast
- 6 ounces scrambled tofu with spinach and 1 slice whole-grain toast (protein, slow-burning carbs, fiber)

Snack
- ½ cup low-fat cottage cheese with peaches (protein, calcium)

Lunch
- Grilled shrimp (4) salad with mixed greens, avocado, and a citrus vinaigrette (protein, omega-3s)

Snack
- 1 cup celery and carrot sticks with 2 tablespoons hummus (fiber, magnesium)

Dinner
- 2 cups beef stir-fry with broccoli, snap peas, and ½ cup brown rice (protein, iron)

Snack
- 1 medium apple with 1 tablespoon almond butter (antioxidants, fiber, monounsaturated fats)

DAY 6

Breakfast
- 8-ounce Greek yogurt parfait with mixed berries and granola (protein, calcium, fiber)

Snack
- 1 to 2 hard-boiled eggs with seasoning of your choice (protein, vitamin B_6)

Lunch
- Black bean and sweet potato burrito with a side of salsa (protein, fiber, vitamin B_9)

Snack
- 20 cashews (magnesium, healthy fats)

Dinner
- 6 ounces grilled mackerel with ½ cup quinoa and ½ cup sautéed Swiss chard (protein, omega-3s, calcium)

Snack
- 1 cup of fortified almond milk (calcium, fiber, protein)

DAY 7

Breakfast
- 2 small whole-grain waffles (6-inch diameter) with strawberries and a dollop of low-fat yogurt (fiber, slow-burning carbs, vitamin B_9, calcium)

Snack
- 1 cup edamame (protein, magnesium, iron)

Lunch
- Turkey and avocado wrap with a side of mixed greens (protein, fiber)

Snack
- 10-ounce green smoothie with spinach, banana, and fortified almond milk (fiber, magnesium, protein, calcium, vitamin B_6)

Dinner
- 6-ounce grilled or baked boneless, skinless chicken breast with ½ cup quinoa and steamed broccoli (protein, slow-burning carbs, vitamin B_6, calcium)

Snack
- 4 small squares of dark chocolate (iron, magnesium, antioxidants)

DAY 8

Breakfast
- 2 scrambled eggs with smoked salmon and 1 whole-grain English muffin (protein, slow-burning carbs, omega-3s)

Snack
- 10-ounce smoothie with kale, banana, chia seeds, and fortified almond milk (calcium, fiber, magnesium, protein)

Lunch
- 2 cups quinoa salad with chickpeas, cucumbers, and tomatoes (protein, slow-burning carbs, fiber, vitamin B_6)

Snack
- 20 walnuts (omega-3s, magnesium)

Dinner
- 6 ounces grilled chicken with a side of ½ cup spinach, ½ cup brown rice, and ½ cup roasted beets (protein, iron, fiber)

Snack
- 6 ounces low-fat yogurt with 1 teaspoon honey (protein, calcium, vitamin B_6)

DAY 9

Breakfast
- 8-ounce Greek yogurt parfait with mixed berries and granola (protein, calcium, fiber)

Snack
- 1 to 2 hard-boiled eggs with seasoning of your choice (protein, vitamin B$_6$)

Lunch
- Black bean and sweet potato burrito with a side of salsa (protein, fiber, vitamin B$_9$)

Snack
- 20 cashews (magnesium, monounsaturated fats)

Dinner
- 6 ounces grilled mackerel with ½ cup quinoa and ½ cup sautéed Swiss chard (protein, omega-3s, calcium)

Snack
- 1 cup of fortified almond milk (calcium, fiber, protein)

DAY 10

Breakfast
- 2 small whole-grain waffles (6-inch diameter) with strawberries and a dollop of low-fat yogurt (fiber, vitamin B$_9$, slow-burning carbs, calcium)

Snack
- 1 cup edamame (protein, magnesium, iron)

Lunch
- Turkey and avocado wrap with a side of mixed greens (protein, fiber)

Snack
- 10-ounce green smoothie with spinach, banana, and fortified almond milk (calcium, fiber, magnesium, vitamin B$_6$)

Dinner
- 6-ounce grilled boneless, skinless chicken breast with quinoa and steamed broccoli (protein, vitamin B$_6$, calcium)

Snack
- 4 small squares dark chocolate (iron, magnesium, antioxidants)

DAY 11

Breakfast
- 6 ounces scrambled tofu with spinach and whole-grain toast (protein, slow-burning carbs, fiber)

Snack
- ½ cup low-fat cottage cheese with peaches (protein, calcium)

Lunch
- Grilled shrimp (4) salad with mixed greens, ½ small avocado, and a citrus vinaigrette (protein, omega-3s)

Snack
- 1 cup celery and carrot sticks with 2 tablespoons hummus (fiber, protein, magnesium)

Dinner
- 2 cups beef stir-fry with broccoli, snap peas, and ½ cup brown rice (protein, slow-burning carbs, iron)

Snack
- 1 medium apple with 1 tablespoon almond butter (antioxidants, fiber, monounsaturated fats)

DAY 12

Breakfast
- 1½ cups oatmeal with flaxseeds, blueberries, and a dollop of Greek yogurt (fiber, omega-3s, protein, slow-burning carbs, calcium)

Snack
- ½ cup cottage cheese with pineapple (calcium, iron, magnesium, protein, vitamin B_6)

Lunch
- 1½ cups lentil and vegetable soup with a side of mixed greens (protein, fiber, vitamin B_9)

Snack
- ½ cup mixed nuts (fiber, magnesium, monounsaturated fats, protein)

Dinner
- 6 ounces grilled salmon with ½ cup quinoa and 4 medium roasted asparagus spears (omega-3s, slow-burning carbs, protein, fiber)

Snack
- 1 cup whole-grain pasta with pesto sauce (fiber, protein, slow-burning carbs)

DAY 13

Breakfast
- 2 scrambled eggs with sautéed spinach, whole-grain toast, and a sprinkle of nutritional yeast (protein, slow-burning carbs, vitamin B_6, vitamin B_9)

Snack
- 10-ounce smoothie with kale, banana, chia seeds, and almond milk (calcium, magnesium, protein, fiber)

Lunch
- Turkey and avocado salad with mixed greens and a balsamic vinaigrette (protein, healthy fats, fiber)

Snack
- 1 sliced bell pepper with 2 tablespoons hummus (antioxidants, fiber, protein, vitamin B_6, vitamin B_9)

Dinner
- 6-ounce grilled boneless, skinless chicken breast with ½ cup quinoa and ½ cup steamed broccoli (protein, iron, slow-burning carbs, calcium)

Snack
- 6 ounces low-fat yogurt with honey (protein, calcium)

DAY 14

Breakfast
- 2 small whole-grain pancakes (6-inch diameter) with 1 tablespoon almond butter and mixed berries (fiber, slow-burning carbs, protein)

Snack
- 1 to 2 hard-boiled eggs with seasoning of your choice (protein, vitamin B_6)

Lunch
- 1½ cups chickpea and vegetable curry with ½ cup brown rice (protein, fiber, slow-burning carbs, vitamin B_9)

Snack
- 20 cashews (magnesium, monounsaturated fats)

Dinner
- 6 ounces baked cod with ½ cup quinoa and 1 cup steamed Brussels sprouts (protein, omega-3s, slow-burning carbs, fiber)

Snack
- 1 cup of fortified almond milk (calcium, fiber, protein)

DAY 15

Breakfast
- 6 ounces scrambled tofu with sautéed kale and whole-grain toast (protein, fiber, calcium)

Snack
- ½ cup low-fat cottage cheese with sliced peaches (protein, vitamin B_6)

Lunch
- Grilled shrimp (4) with ½ cup quinoa and ½ cup roasted bell pepper slices (antioxidants, fiber, protein, slow-burning carbs, vitamin B_6, vitamin B_9)

Snack
- 1 cup baby carrots and cucumber slices with 2 tablespoons hummus (fiber, vitamin B_6)

Dinner
- 6-ounce baked boneless, skinless chicken breast with ½ cup brown rice and ½ cup steamed green beans (protein, slow-burning carbs)

Snack
- 1 cup whole-grain pasta with tomato sauce (fiber, slow-burning carbs, iron)

DAY 16

Breakfast
- 2 scrambled eggs with spinach and tomatoes (protein, vitamin B_6, fiber)
- 1 slice whole-grain toast (slow-burning carbs)
- 1 cup orange juice (vitamin B_9)

Lunch
- 6-ounce grilled boneless, skinless chicken chicken breast with 2 cups mixed greens and ¼ cup nuts (protein, vitamin B_6, magnesium, omega-3s)
- ½ cup quinoa (slow-burning carbs)
- ½ cup low-fat yogurt (calcium)

Snack
- ½ cup Greek yogurt with berries and honey (protein, calcium, vitamin B_6)
- 10 almonds (magnesium)

Dinner
- 6 ounces baked or grilled salmon (omega-3s, protein)
- ½ cup brown rice (slow-burning carbs, magnesium)
- 1 cup mixed vegetables (fiber, iron)

Snack
- 1 cup carrot and cucumber sticks and 2 tablespoons hummus (protein, fiber)

DAY 17

Breakfast
- 1½ cups oatmeal with ½ small banana, sliced, and ¼ cup almonds (fiber, protein, slow-burning carbs, monounsaturated fats)

Lunch
- 1½ cups lentil soup with a side salad of greens, chickpeas, and sunflower seeds (fiber, protein, monounsaturated fats, polyunsaturated fats

Snack
- ½ cup mixed berries and 10 cashews (antioxidants, monounsaturated fats)

Dinner
- Grilled tofu with broccoli and brown rice (protein, fiber, iron, magnesium, vitamin B$_6$)

Snack
- 1 small cucumber, sliced, with 2 tablespoons hummus (fiber, protein)

DAY 18

Breakfast
- 2 scrambled eggs with spinach, whole-grain toast, and a side of avocado (protein, fiber, slow-burning carbs, monounsaturated fats)

Snack
- 10-ounce smoothie with kale, banana, chia seeds, and fortified almond milk (calcium, fiber, magnesium, protein)

Lunch
- Turkey and avocado wrap with a side salad (protein, fiber, vitamin B$_6$)

Snack
- 1 cup celery and carrot sticks with 2 tablespoons hummus (protein, fiber, vitamin B$_6$)

Dinner
- 2 cups beef stir-fry with ½ cup quinoa and ½ cup sautéed bok choy (protein, iron, slow-burning carbs, calcium)

Snack
- 1 sliced apple with 1 tablespoon almond butter (antioxidants, fiber, monounsaturated fats)

DAY 19

Breakfast
- 2 small whole-grain pancakes (6-inch diameter) with fresh berries, 1 tablespoon almond butter, and maple syrup (fiber, protein, slow-burning carbs, iron)

Snack
- 1 cup edamame (protein, calcium, vitamin B_6, vitamin B_9, omega-3s, magnesium, fiber, iron, whole grains)

Lunch
- Turkey and avocado wrap with a side salad of mixed greens (protein, fiber, monounsaturated fats)

Snack
- ½ cup low-fat yogurt with sliced almonds and honey (protein, calcium, magnesium)

Dinner
- Grilled shrimp (6) with ½ cup quinoa and ½ cup sautéed kale (protein, magnesium, slow-burning carbs, fiber)

Snack
- Pumpkin seeds (pepitas) and dark chocolate chips (½ cup total) (protein, calcium, vitamin B_6, vitamin B_9, omega-3s, magnesium, antioxidants, fiber, iron, whole grains)

DAY 20

Breakfast
- 8-ounce Greek yogurt parfait with strawberries, honey, and granola (protein, calcium, vitamin B_6)

Snack
- 1 to 2 hard-boiled eggs with seasoning of your choice (protein, vitamin B_6)

Lunch
- 1½ cups lentil and vegetable stir-fry with brown rice (protein, fiber, slow-burning carbs, magnesium)

Snack
- A handful of almonds (magnesium, monounsaturated fats)

Dinner
- 6 ounces grilled salmon with ½ cup quinoa and ½ cup steamed broccoli (omega-3s, protein, magnesium, vitamin B$_6$, calcium)

Snack
- 1 cup of fortified almond milk (calcium, fiber, protein)

DAY 21

Breakfast
- 1½ cups oatmeal with 1 tablespoon flaxseeds, mixed berries, and a dollop of Greek yogurt (fiber, omega-3s, protein, slow-burning carbs, calcium)

Snack
- ½ cup cottage cheese with pineapple (calcium, iron, magnesium, protein, vitamin B$_6$)

Lunch
- 1½ cups lentil and vegetable soup with a side of mixed greens (protein, fiber, vitamin B$_6$)

Snack
- ½ cup mixed nuts such as Brazil nuts, almonds, cashews, pecans, and peanuts (fiber, magnesium, monounsaturated fats, protein)

Dinner
- 6 ounces grilled salmon with ½ cup quinoa and 4 medium roasted asparagus spears (omega-3s, protein, fiber)

Snack
- 1 cup whole-grain pasta with a tomato and basil sauce (fiber, slow-burning carbs, iron)

DAY 22

Breakfast

- 2 scrambled eggs with spinach, whole-grain toast, and a side of avocado (protein, fiber, slow-burning carbs, monounsaturated fats)

Snack

- 10-ounce smoothie with kale, banana, chia seeds, and fortified almond milk (calcium, fiber, magnesium, protein)

Lunch

- Turkey and avocado wrap with a side salad (protein, fiber, monounsaturated fats, vitamin B_6)

Snack

- 1 cup celery and carrot sticks with 2 tablespoons hummus (fiber, protein, vitamin B_6)

Dinner

- 2 cups beef stir-fry with ½ cup quinoa and sautéed bok choy (protein, fiber, iron, slow-burning carbs, calcium)

Snack

- 1 sliced apple with almond butter (antioxidants, fiber, monounsaturated fats)

DAY 23

Breakfast

- 1½ cups oatmeal with flaxseeds, mixed berries, and a dollop of Greek yogurt (fiber, omega-3s, protein, slow-burning carbs, calcium)

Snack

- ½ cup cottage cheese with pineapple (calcium, iron, magnesium, protein, vitamin B_6)

Lunch

- 1½ cups lentil and vegetable soup with a side of mixed greens (protein, fiber, vitamin B_6)

Snack
- ½ cup mixed nuts (fiber, magnesium, monounsaturated fats, protein)

Dinner
- 6 ounces grilled salmon with quinoa and roasted asparagus (omega-3s, protein, slow-burning carbs, fiber)

Snack
- 1 cup whole-grain pasta with a tomato and basil sauce (fiber, protein, slow-burning carbs, iron)

DAY 24

Breakfast
- 2 small whole-grain pancakes (6-inch diameter) with 1 tablespoon almond butter and mixed berries (fiber, monounsaturated fats, slow-burning carbs, protein)

Snack
- 1 to 2 hard-boiled eggs with seasoning of your choice (protein, vitamin B_6)

Lunch
- 1½ cups chickpea and vegetable curry with brown rice (protein, fiber, slow-burning carbs, vitamin B_9)

Snack
- 20 cashews (magnesium, monounsaturated fats)

Dinner
- 6 ounces baked or grilled cod with ½ cup quinoa and 1 cup roasted Brussels sprouts (protein, omega-3s, fiber)

Snack
- 1 cup of fortified almond milk (calcium, fiber, protein)

DAY 25

Breakfast
- 8-ounce Greek yogurt parfait with mixed berries and granola (protein, calcium, fiber)

Snack
- 1 to 2 hard-boiled eggs with seasoning of your choice (protein, vitamin B_6)

Lunch
- Black bean and sweet potato burrito with a side of salsa (protein, fiber, vitamin B_9)

Snack
- 20 cashews (magnesium, monounsaturated fats)

Dinner
- 6 ounces grilled mackerel with quinoa and sautéed Swiss chard (protein, omega-3s, calcium)

Snack
- 1 cup edamame (protein, magnesium)

DAY 26

Breakfast
- 2 small whole-grain pancakes (6-inch diameter) with 1 tablespoon almond butter and mixed berries (antioxidants, fiber, slow-burning carbs, protein)

Snack
- 1 to 2 hard-boiled eggs with seasoning of your choice (protein, vitamin B_6)

Lunch
- 1½ cups chickpea and ½ cup vegetable curry with ½ cup brown rice (protein, fiber, vitamin B_9)

Snack
- 20 cashews (magnesium, monounsaturated fats)

Dinner
- 6 ounces baked cod with ½ cup quinoa and 1 cup roasted Brussels sprouts (protein, omega-3s, slow-burning carbs, fiber)

Snack
- 1 sliced apple with 1 tablespoon almond butter (antioxidants, fiber, monounsaturated fats)

DAY 27

Breakfast
- 1½ cups oatmeal with 1 tablespoon flaxseeds, mixed berries, and a dollop of Greek yogurt (fiber, omega-3s, protein, slow-burning carbs, calcium)

Snack
- ½ cup cottage cheese with pineapple (calcium, iron, magnesium, protein, vitamin B_6)

Lunch
- 1½ cups lentil and vegetable soup with a side of mixed greens (protein, fiber, vitamin B_6)

Snack
- ½ cup mixed nuts such as Brazil nuts, almonds, cashews, pecans, and peanuts (fiber, magnesium, monounsaturated fats, protein)

Dinner
- 6 ounces grilled salmon with ½ cup quinoa and 4 medium roasted asparagus spears (omega-3s, protein, slow-burning carbs, fiber)

Snack
- 1 cup whole-grain pasta with a tomato and basil sauce (fiber, protein, slow-burning carbs, iron)

DAY 28

Breakfast
- 8-ounce Greek yogurt parfait with strawberries, honey, and granola (protein, calcium, vitamin B_6)

Snack
- 1 to 2 hard-boiled eggs with seasoning of your choice (protein, vitamin B_6)

Lunch
- 1½ cups lentil and 1 cup vegetable stir-fry with ½ cup brown rice (protein, fiber, magnesium, slow-burning carbs)

Snack
- 20 almonds (magnesium, monounsaturated fats)

Dinner
- 6 ounces grilled salmon with ½ cup quinoa and ½ cup steamed broccoli (omega-3s, protein, slow-burning carbs, calcium)

Snack
- 4 small squares dark chocolate (iron, magnesium, antioxidants)

DAY 29

Breakfast
- 2 scrambled eggs with sautéed spinach, whole-grain toast, and a side of avocado (monounsaturated fats, protein, fiber, slow-burning carbs, vitamin B_6)

Snack
- ½ cup low-fat cottage cheese with sliced peaches (protein, calcium)

Lunch
- Grilled shrimp (6) with quinoa and roasted bell peppers (antioxidants, fiber, protein, slow-burning carbs, vitamin B_6, vitamin B_9)

Snack
- 1 cup baby carrots and cucumber slices with 2 tablespoons hummus (fiber, vitamin B_6)

Dinner
- 6 ounces grilled chicken with ½ cup brown rice and ½ cup steamed green beans (protein, slow-burning carbs)

Snack
- 6 ounces low-fat yogurt with honey (antioxidants, protein, calcium)

DAY 30

Breakfast
- 2 small whole-grain pancakes (6-inch diameter) with 1 tablespoon almond butter and mixed berries (fiber, monounsaturated fats, protein, slow-burning carbs)

Snack
- 1 to 2 hard-boiled eggs with seasoning of your choice (protein, vitamin B_6)

Lunch
- 1½ cups chickpea and vegetable curry with brown rice (protein, fiber, vitamin B_9)

Snack
- 20 cashews (magnesium, monounsaturated fats)

Dinner
- 6 ounces baked or grilled cod with ½ cup quinoa and 1 cup roasted Brussels sprouts (protein, omega-3s, fiber)

Evening Snack
- 1 cup of fortified almond milk (calcium, fiber, protein)

THE 40s

This is an important decade that can be instrumental in determining not only how long but also how well you live. These are the years when what you've eaten and how you've treated your body will be reflected in your health. Conditions such as high blood pressure, obesity, and even some forms of heart disease can manifest in this decade, as well as muscle and bone loss from poor nutrition and insufficient or ineffective exercise. However, you can make significant strides through your nutrition. Increasing your antioxidants to fight disease, upping your calcium to protect your bones, and eating more monounsaturated fats to prevent the clogging of your arteries are just a few measures you can take to increase your odds of a healthier decade. Remember, eat well to live well.

Below you will find some samples of different meals and snacks that incorporate the top 10 power nutrients for your decade. The quantity for each nutrient will depend on how much of the different foods you consume. There are numerous online nutrient calculators that will allow you to input the ingredients of the meals and give you an approximation of the nutrient quantities. Remember, these are only samples to give you an idea. There are infinite combinations of foods and recipes that you can choose from that will supply you with various nutrients. It would not be possible to include them all in one book, let alone a single chapter.

BREAKFAST

- 8 ounces Greek yogurt with berries (antioxidants, calcium, vitamin B_{12}), 1 tablespoon chia seeds (antioxidants, calcium, fiber, iron, magnesium, omega-3s), 20 almonds (1 ounce) (monounsaturated fats, magnesium)
- 1½ cups oatmeal with ½ small banana, sliced (fiber, potassium, protein, iron)
- 2 scrambled eggs (protein, vitamin B_{12}), 1 cup spinach (antioxidants, fiber, calcium, iron, magnesium, potassium), ½ avocado, sliced (antioxidants, monounsaturated fats, fiber, magnesium)
- 1 cup cottage cheese (protein, calcium), 1 cup mixed berries (antioxidants, fiber), 1 tablespoon flaxseeds (fiber, magnesium, omega-3s)
- 3 ounces smoked salmon and 1 tablespoon cream cheese on 1 slice whole-grain toast (omega-3s, protein, slow-burning carbs, vitamin D, calcium), 1 sliced kiwi (vitamin C, potassium)
- 8-ounce Greek yogurt parfait with mixed berries (antioxidants, calcium, vitamin B_{12}), 1 tablespoon almond butter (monounsaturated fats), ¼ cup whole-grain granola (fiber, protein, iron, slow-burning carbs, vitamin D)
- 6 ounces scrambled tofu with spinach and tomatoes (antioxidants, fiber, calcium, iron, magnesium, potassium, protein), 1 orange, sliced (vitamin C, antioxidants)

- 2 whole-grain waffles with fresh blueberries (antioxidants, fiber), ½ cup Greek yogurt (calcium, slow-burning carbs, vitamin B_{12})
- 2-egg spinach and mushroom omelet (antioxidants, fiber, calcium, iron, magnesium, potassium, protein), 1 slice whole-grain toast (fiber), 1 sliced orange (antioxidants, slow-burning carbs, vitamin C)
- 12-ounce smoothie with kale, banana, chia seeds, and fortified almond milk (antioxidants, calcium, fiber, iron, magnesium, omega-3s, protein, vitamin D), and ¼ cup whole-grain granola (iron, slow-burning carbs, vitamin D)
- 8-ounce Greek yogurt parfait with 1 teaspoon honey and mixed berries (antioxidants, calcium, fiber, vitamin B_{12}), 1 ounce walnuts (monounsaturated fats, magnesium)
- 2 scrambled eggs with sautéed spinach and feta cheese (antioxidants, fiber, calcium, iron, magnesium, potassium, protein)
- 1 cup overnight oats with ½ small banana, sliced, and 1 tablespoon almond butter (potassium, monounsaturated fats), 1 tablespoon chia seeds (antioxidants, calcium, fiber, iron, magnesium, omega-3s, slow-burning carbs)
- 12-ounce smoothie with kale, pineapple, flaxseeds, and coconut milk (antioxidants, potassium, omega-3s), ¼ cup whole-grain granola (protein, iron, vitamin D, slow-burning carbs)
- 6 ounces scrambled tofu with bell peppers and tomatoes (protein, iron, antioxidants), 1 slice whole-grain toast (fiber), ½ cup sliced strawberries (antioxidants, fiber, potassium, slow-burning carbs)
- 8 ounces Greek yogurt with 1 teaspoon honey and sliced peaches (antioxidants, calcium, vitamin B_{12}), 20 almonds (monounsaturated fats, magnesium)
- 1½ cups overnight oats with sliced strawberries and 1 tablespoon almond butter (antioxidants, fiber, potassium, slow-burning carbs, monounsaturated fats), 1 tablespoon chia seeds (antioxidants, calcium, fiber, iron, magnesium, omega-3s)
- 12-ounce green smoothie with kale, pineapple, flaxseeds, and

fortified almond milk (antioxidants, calcium, fiber, iron, magnesium, omega-3s, vitamin D), ¼ cup whole-grain granola (protein, iron, vitamin D)

- 2 scrambled eggs with sautéed spinach and tomatoes (antioxidants, fiber, calcium, iron, magnesium, potassium, protein, vitamin B_{12}), 1 slice whole-grain toast (fiber), 1 sliced kiwi (vitamin C, slow-burning carbs, antioxidants)
- 8 ounces Greek yogurt with 1 teaspoon honey and sliced peaches (antioxidants, calcium, vitamin B_{12}), 20 almonds (monounsaturated fats, magnesium)
- 2 scrambled eggs with sautéed mushrooms and spinach (antioxidants, fiber, calcium, iron, magnesium, potassium, protein, vitamin B_{12}), 1 slice whole-grain toast (fiber), 1 cup strawberries (antioxidants, fiber, potassium, slow-burning carbs)

LUNCH

- Turkey and avocado wrap with mixed greens in a whole-grain tortilla (protein, monounsaturated fats, fiber, antioxidants, magnesium)
- 2 cups chickpea and vegetable stir-fry with tofu (iron, magnesium, protein), 1 cup spinach and kale salad (antioxidants, fiber, calcium, iron, magnesium, potassium, protein, vitamin B_{12})
- 2 cups quinoa and black bean salad with a lime vinaigrette (iron, magnesium), 1 cup mixed greens (calcium, antioxidants)
- 2 cups chickpea and vegetable salad with a tahini dressing (iron, magnesium, protein), 1 cup spinach and kale salad (antioxidants, fiber, calcium, iron, magnesium, potassium)
- 2 cups turkey and avocado salad with mixed greens (protein, monounsaturated fats, antioxidants, fiber, magnesium), whole-grain pita (fiber, iron, magnesium, slow-burning carbs)
- 2 cups lentil and vegetable stir-fry (fiber, iron, magnesium, potassium), 1 cup spinach and kale salad (antioxidants, fiber, calcium, iron, magnesium, potassium)
- 2 cups quinoa salad with roasted vegetables and a balsamic vin-

aigrette (fiber, magnesium, antioxidants), 1 cup mixed greens (calcium, fiber, iron)

- 2 cups grilled shrimp and quinoa bowl with mixed vegetables (protein, magnesium, B vitamins)
- 2 cups lentil and vegetable soup (fiber, iron, magnesium, potassium), 1 cup spinach and kale salad (antioxidants, fiber, calcium, iron, magnesium, potassium)
- 2 cups chickpea and vegetable curry (iron, magnesium, protein), ½ cup cooked quinoa (magnesium, slow-burning carbs, vitamin B_6, vitamin B_9, vitamin B_{12})
- 2 cups quinoa salad with chickpeas, cucumbers, and a lemon-tahini dressing (fiber, iron, magnesium, protein, slow-burning carbs), 1 cup mixed greens (calcium, antioxidants)
- 2 cups grilled chicken Caesar salad (fiber, protein, calcium, magnesium)
- 1½ cups quinoa and black bean salad with a lime vinaigrette (iron, magnesium, slow-burning carbs), 1 cup spinach and arugula salad with ¼ cup pecans (antioxidants, fiber, calcium, iron, magnesium, monounsaturated fats, potassium), 1 orange, sliced (antioxidants, vitamin C)
- Turkey and avocado wrap in whole-grain tortilla (protein, monounsaturated fats, fiber, antioxidants, fiber, magnesium, slow-burning carbs), 2 cups mixed greens salad (antioxidants, fiber), 1 cup sweet potato fries (iron, potassium)

DINNER

- 1½ cups chickpea and vegetable stir-fry with 1 cup cooked brown rice (fiber, iron, magnesium, potassium, slow-burning carbs, vitamin B_6)
- 6 ounces baked or grilled cod with 1 cup chopped asparagus, and 1 cup mashed sweet potatoes (iron, magnesium, omega-3s, potassium, vitamin B_{12}, vitamin D)
- 6 ounces grilled tofu with 1 cup steamed kale and ½ cup cooked

quinoa (calcium, fiber, iron, magnesium, protein, slow-burning carbs, vitamin B_6, vitamin B_9, vitamin B_{12})

- 6-ounce grilled boneless, skinless chicken breast with mango salsa, 1 cup steamed broccoli, and 1 cup wild rice (calcium, fiber, iron, magnesium, protein, vitamin B_6, vitamin B_9, vitamin C)

- 6 ounces baked trout with 1 cup roasted Brussels sprouts and ½ cup cooked quinoa (fiber, iron, magnesium, potassium, protein, omega-3s, slow-burning carbs, vitamin B_6, vitamin B_9, vitamin B_{12}, vitamin D)

- 6 ounces grilled swordfish with 1 cup sautéed Swiss chard and 1 cup cooked brown rice (calcium, fiber, magnesium, omega-3s, potassium, protein, slow-burning carbs, vitamin B_6)

- 6 ounces baked cod with a lemon-herb sauce, 1 cup chopped roasted asparagus, and ½ cup cooked quinoa (fiber, iron, magnesium, omega-3s, potassium, slow-burning carbs, vitamin B_6, vitamin B_9, vitamin B_{12}, vitamin D)

- 6 ounces grilled salmon with dill sauce with 1 cup sautéed spinach and 1 cup cooked brown or white rice (antioxidants, calcium, fiber, iron, magnesium, omega-3s, potassium, protein, vitamin B_6, vitamin D)

- 6 ounces grilled salmon with dill sauce with 1 cup sautéed spinach and 1 cup cooked brown rice (antioxidants, calcium, fiber, iron, magnesium, omega-3s, potassium, protein, slow-burning carbs, vitamin B_6, vitamin D)

- 6 ounces grilled tilapia with 1 cup roasted Brussels sprouts and 1 cup brown or white rice (fiber, iron, magnesium, potassium, protein, vitamin B_6, vitamin D)

- 6 ounces grilled swordfish with mango salsa, 1 cup steamed Swiss chard, and 1 cup cooked brown rice (calcium, fiber, magnesium, omega-3s, potassium, protein, slow-burning carbs, vitamin B_6)

- 6 ounces grilled salmon with a lemon-dill sauce with 4 medium roasted asparagus spears and ½ cup cooked quinoa (fiber, iron, magnesium, omega-3s, potassium, protein, slow-burning carbs, vitamin B_6, vitamin B_9, vitamin B_{12}, vitamin D)

- 6-ounce baked or grilled boneless, skinless chicken breast with rosemary, 1 cup sautéed spinach, and 1 cup cooked brown rice (antioxidants, calcium, fiber, iron, magnesium, potassium, protein, slow-burning carbs, vitamin B_{12})
- 6 ounces baked trout with a lemon-herb sauce with 1 cup roasted Brussels sprouts and 1 cup cooked brown rice (fiber, iron, magnesium, potassium, protein, omega-3s, slow-burning carbs, vitamin B_6, vitamin D)
- 6 ounces grilled tilapia with 1 cup steamed Swiss chard and ½ cup cooked quinoa (calcium, fiber, magnesium, potassium, protein, slow-burning carbs, vitamin B_6, vitamin B_9, vitamin B_{12}, vitamin D)
- 6 ounces grilled or baked salmon with a garlic herb sauce, 1 cup steamed broccoli, and 1 cup cooked brown or white rice (calcium, fiber, iron, magnesium, omega-3s, protein, vitamin B_6, vitamin D)
- 6-ounce grilled boneless, skinless chicken breast with a lemon-herb marinade, 1 cup sautéed spinach, and ½ cup cooked quinoa (antioxidants, calcium, fiber, iron, magnesium, potassium, protein, slow-burning carbs, vitamin B_6, vitamin B_9, vitamin B_{12})

SNACKS

- Almonds (20) (monounsaturated fats, calcium, magnesium, antioxidants)
- Chia pudding (½ cup) with 1 tablespoon chia seeds (antioxidants, calcium, fiber, iron, magnesium, omega-3s)
- Greek yogurt (½ cup) with mixed berries (½ cup) (antioxidants, calcium, vitamin D)
- Spinach and kale chips (1½ cups) (iron, calcium, antioxidants)
- Dark chocolate (1.5 ounces, 85% cocoa) (iron, magnesium, antioxidants)
- Edamame (1 cup of pods) (antioxidants, calcium, magnesium, protein)

- Sardines (in extra-virgin olive oil, 1 small tin) (omega-3s, vitamin B_{12}, potassium, protein)
- Pumpkin seeds (¼ cup) (magnesium, iron, antioxidants)
- Quinoa salad (1 cup) (iron, magnesium, slow-burning carbs, vitamin B_{12})
- Blueberries (1½ cups) (antioxidants, fiber, vitamin C)
- Avocado slices (½ avocado) (monounsaturated fats, potassium, magnesium)
- Muesli with almonds and flaxseeds (½ cup serving) (omega-3s, magnesium, protein)
- Swiss chard wraps with hummus (2 wraps) (iron, calcium, antioxidants)
- Broccoli florets (2 cups, steamed) (calcium, iron, vitamin C)
- Almond butter (1 tablespoon) with apple slices (1 medium apple) (monounsaturated fats, antioxidants)
- Sunflower seeds (¼ cup) (magnesium, iron)
- Brazil nuts (about 3 nuts) (selenium, magnesium)
- Canned tuna (in extra-virgin olive oil, 1 can, typically around 5 ounces) (omega-3s, vitamin D, vitamin B_{12}, potassium)
- Oranges (2 medium oranges) (antioxidants, vitamin C)
- Green tea (1 cup, unsweetened) (antioxidants, vitamin D)

Now that you have some examples of the types of meals and snacks you can eat and the power nutrients they contain, you can mix and match them to create daily meal plans. Below, you will find menus with approximately 2,000 to 2,500 calories per day, but if you want to eat less, you can adjust for a lower calorie count. This is meant to be a stress-free, flexible plan that you will enjoy. You can make reasonable substitutions such as swapping brown rice for quinoa and vice versa. You can mix days by taking meals or snacks from one day and substituting it in another day. For example, if you don't have the ingredients for dinner on day 2, but you have the ingredients for dinner on day 7, then you can have the day 7 dinner on day 2. The idea is to get as much of your top 10 power nutrients into your diet as possible and have fun while doing it.

30-DAY MEAL PLAN

DAY 1

Breakfast
- 8 ounces Greek yogurt with berries (antioxidants, calcium, vitamin B_{12})
- 1 tablespoon chia seeds (antioxidants, calcium, fiber, iron, magnesium, omega-3s)
- 20 almonds (1 ounce) (monounsaturated fats, magnesium)

Lunch
- 6 ounces grilled salmon (omega-3s, protein, vitamin D)
- 2 cups spinach salad (antioxidants, fiber, calcium, iron, magnesium, potassium)
- ½ cup cooked quinoa (fiber, magnesium, slow-burning carbs, vitamin B_6, vitamin B_9, vitamin B_{12})

Snack
- 1 cup carrot sticks (antioxidants, iron, calcium, potassium)

Dinner
- 1½ cups chickpea and vegetable stir-fry (iron, magnesium, potassium)
- 1 cup cooked brown rice (fiber, magnesium, vitamin B_6)

DAY 2

Breakfast
- 1½ cups oatmeal with sliced bananas (slow-burning carbs, potassium, iron)
- ¼ cup walnuts (monounsaturated fats)

Lunch
- 6-ounce grilled boneless, skinless chicken breast (protein)
- 2 cups spinach and kale salad (antioxidants, fiber, calcium, iron, magnesium, potassium)
- ½ cup cooked quinoa (fiber, magnesium, slow-burning carbs, vitamin B_6, vitamin B_9, vitamin B_{12})

Snack
- 1 cup blueberries (antioxidants, vitamin C)

Dinner
- 6 ounces baked or grilled cod (omega-3s, vitamin D)
- 1 cup asparagus (iron, potassium)
- 1 cup mashed sweet potatoes (magnesium, vitamin B_{12})

DAY 3

Breakfast
- 2 scrambled eggs (protein, vitamin B_{12})
- 1 cup spinach (antioxidants, fiber, calcium, iron, magnesium, potassium)
- ½ avocado, sliced (antioxidants, monounsaturated fats, fiber, magnesium)

Lunch
- 2 cups lentil soup (fiber, iron, magnesium, potassium, protein)
- 2 cups mixed greens salad (antioxidants, calcium, fiber, iron, magnesium)
- ½ cup cooked quinoa (fiber, magnesium, slow-burning carbs, vitamin B_6, vitamin B_9, vitamin B_{12})

Snack
- 1 cup strawberries (antioxidants, fiber, potassium)

Dinner
- 6 grilled shrimp (protein, vitamin D)
- 1 cup broccoli (calcium, fiber, iron, magnesium)
- 1 cup cooked brown rice (fiber, magnesium, slow-burning carbs, vitamin B_6)

DAY 4

Breakfast
- 1 cup cottage cheese (protein, calcium)
- 1 cup mixed berries (antioxidants, fiber)
- 1 tablespoon flaxseeds (fiber, omega-3s, magnesium)

Lunch
- Turkey and avocado wrap in whole-grain tortilla (protein, monounsaturated fats, fiber, antioxidants, magnesium)
- 2 cups mixed greens salad (antioxidants, fiber)
- 1 cup sweet potato fries (iron, potassium)

Snack
- 20 almonds (monounsaturated fats, magnesium)

Dinner
- 6 ounces grilled tofu (protein)
- 1 cup steamed kale (calcium, iron)
- ½ cup cooked quinoa (fiber, magnesium, slow-burning carbs, vitamin B_6, vitamin B_9, vitamin B_{12})

DAY 5

Breakfast
- 3 ounces smoked salmon and 1 tablespoon cream cheese on whole-grain toast (omega-3s, protein, vitamin D, calcium, slow-burning carbs)
- 1 kiwi, sliced (vitamin C, potassium)

Lunch
- 1½ cups quinoa and black bean salad with a lime vinaigrette (fiber, iron, magnesium, slow-burning carbs)
- 1 cup spinach and arugula salad with ¼ cup pecans (antioxidants, fiber, calcium, iron, magnesium, monounsaturated fats, potassium)
- 1 orange, sliced (antioxidants, vitamin C)

Snack
- 1 cup carrot and cucumber sticks with ¼ cup guacamole (monounsaturated fats, fiber, antioxidants, iron, calcium, potassium)

Dinner
- 6-ounce grilled boneless, skinless chicken breast with mango salsa (protein, vitamin C)
- 1 cup steamed broccoli (calcium, fiber, iron, magnesium)
- 1 cup wild rice (magnesium, B vitamins)

DAY 6

Breakfast
- 8-ounce Greek yogurt parfait with mixed berries (antioxidants, calcium, vitamin B_{12}), 1 tablespoon almond butter (monounsaturated fats, fiber), and ¼ cup whole-grain granola (protein, iron, vitamin D)

Lunch
- 2 cups lentil and vegetable soup (fiber, iron, magnesium, potassium)
- 2 cups spinach and kale salad (antioxidants, fiber, calcium, iron, magnesium, potassium)
- 1 whole-grain roll (fiber)

Snack
- 1 cup sliced red bell peppers with hummus (vitamin C, iron)

Dinner
- 6 ounces baked trout (protein, omega-3s, vitamin D)
- 1 cup roasted Brussels sprouts (iron, potassium)
- ½ cup cooked quinoa (fiber, magnesium, vitamin B_6, vitamin B_9, vitamin B_{12})

DAY 7

Breakfast
- 6 ounces scrambled tofu with spinach and tomatoes (antioxidants, fiber, calcium, iron, magnesium, potassium, protein)
- 1 orange, sliced (vitamin C, antioxidants)

Lunch
- 2 cups turkey and avocado salad with mixed greens (protein, monounsaturated fats, antioxidants, fiber, magnesium)
- 1 whole-grain pita (fiber, iron, magnesium)

Snack
- ½ cup mixed nuts (fiber, monounsaturated fats, magnesium, protein)

Dinner
- 6 ounces grilled swordfish (omega-3s, protein)
- 1 cup sautéed Swiss chard (calcium, potassium)
- 1 cup cooked brown rice (fiber, slow-burning carbs, magnesium, vitamin B_6)

DAY 8

Breakfast
- 2 small or 1 large whole-grain waffle with fresh blueberries (antioxidants, fiber)
- ½ cup Greek yogurt (calcium, slow-burning carbs, vitamin B_{12})

Lunch
- 2 cups Caesar salad with grilled boneless, skinless chicken breast (protein, calcium, magnesium)
- ½ cup whole-grain croutons (fiber)

Snack
- 1 small cucumber, sliced, with 2 tablespoons tzatziki sauce (mono-unsaturated fats, potassium)

Dinner
- 6 ounces baked cod with a lemon-herb sauce (omega-3s, vitamin D)
- 1 cup roasted asparagus (iron, potassium)
- ½ cup cooked quinoa (fiber, magnesium, vitamin B_6, vitamin B_9, vitamin B_{12})

DAY 9

Breakfast
- 2-egg spinach and mushroom omelet (antioxidants, fiber, calcium, iron, magnesium, potassium, protein)
- 1 slice whole-grain toast (fiber)
- 1 sliced orange (vitamin C, antioxidants)

Lunch
- 2 cups quinoa salad with chickpeas, cucumbers, and a lemon-tahini dressing (fiber, iron, magnesium, protein)
- 1 cup mixed greens (calcium, fiber, antioxidants)

Snack
- 1 cup mixed berries (antioxidants, fiber, vitamin C)

Dinner
- 6 ounces grilled salmon with dill sauce (omega-3s, protein, vitamin D)
- 1 cup sautéed spinach (antioxidants, fiber, calcium, iron, magnesium, potassium)
- 1 cup cooked brown rice (fiber, magnesium, vitamin B_6)

DAY 10

Breakfast
- 12-ounce smoothie with kale, banana, chia seeds, and fortified almond milk (antioxidants, calcium, fiber, iron, magnesium, omega-3s, vitamin D)
- ¼ cup whole-grain granola (protein, iron, vitamin D)

Lunch
- Turkey and avocado wrap with mixed greens in a whole-grain tortilla (protein, monounsaturated fats, antioxidants, fiber, magnesium)

Snack
- 1 cup carrot and celery sticks with 2 tablespoons hummus (monounsaturated fats, iron, antioxidants, calcium, potassium)

Dinner
- 6-ounce baked or grilled boneless, skinless chicken breast with rosemary (protein, vitamin B_{12})
- 1 cup steamed broccoli (calcium, fiber, iron, magnesium)
- ½ cup cooked quinoa (fiber, magnesium, slow-burning carbs, vitamin B_6, vitamin B_9, vitamin B_{12})

DAY 11

Breakfast
- 8-ounce Greek yogurt parfait with 1 teaspoon honey, walnuts, and mixed berries (antioxidants, calcium, magnesium, monounsaturated fats, vitamin B_{12})

Lunch
- 2 cups lentil and vegetable stir-fry (iron, magnesium, potassium)
- 1 cup mixed greens salad (antioxidants, fiber)

Snack
- 1 sliced apple with 1 tablespoon almond butter (monounsaturated fats, fiber)

Dinner
- 6 ounces grilled tilapia (protein, vitamin D)
- 1 cup roasted Brussels sprouts (fiber, iron, potassium)
- 1 cup brown or white rice (fiber, magnesium, vitamin B_6)

DAY 12

Breakfast
- 2 scrambled eggs with sautéed spinach and feta cheese (antioxidants, fiber, calcium, iron, magnesium, potassium, protein)
- 1 slice of whole-grain toast (fiber)
- 1 kiwi, sliced (vitamin C, potassium)

Lunch
- 2 cups chickpea and vegetable curry (iron, magnesium, fiber, protein)
- ½ cup cooked quinoa (fiber, magnesium, vitamin B_6, vitamin B_9, vitamin B_{12})

Snack
- 1 cup sliced bell peppers and cucumber with 2 tablespoons hummus (monounsaturated fats, iron)

Dinner
- 6 ounces grilled swordfish with mango salsa (omega-3s, protein)
- 1 cup steamed Swiss chard (calcium, potassium)
- 1 cup cooked brown rice (fiber, magnesium, vitamin B_6)

DAY 13

Breakfast
- 1½ cups overnight oats with ½ small banana, sliced, and 1 tablespoon almond butter (potassium, monounsaturated fats, fiber), 1 tablespoon chia seeds (antioxidants, calcium, fiber, iron, magnesium, omega-3s)

Lunch
- 2 cups turkey and avocado salad with mixed greens (protein, monounsaturated fats, antioxidants, fiber, magnesium)
- 1 whole-grain pita (fiber, iron, magnesium)

Snack
- ¼ cup mixed nuts (fiber, monounsaturated fats, magnesium, proteins)

Dinner
- 6 ounces grilled salmon with a lemon-dill sauce (omega-3s, protein, vitamin D)
- 1 cup roasted asparagus (iron, potassium)
- ½ cup cooked quinoa (fiber, magnesium, vitamin B_6, vitamin B_9, vitamin B_{12})

DAY 14

Breakfast
- 12-ounce smoothie with kale, pineapple, flaxseeds, and coconut milk (antioxidants, potassium, omega-3s) and optional ¼ cup whole-grain granola (protein, iron, vitamin D)

Lunch
- 2 cups lentil and vegetable soup (iron, magnesium, potassium)

- 1 cup spinach and kale salad (antioxidants, fiber, calcium, iron, magnesium, potassium)

Snack
- 1 pear, sliced, with 1 tablespoon almond butter (monounsaturated fats, fiber)

Dinner
- 6-ounce baked or grilled boneless, skinless chicken breast with rosemary (protein, vitamin B_{12})
- 1 cup sautéed spinach (antioxidants, fiber, calcium, iron, magnesium, potassium)
- 1 cup cooked brown rice (fiber, magnesium)

DAY 15

Breakfast
- 6 ounces scrambled tofu with bell peppers and tomatoes (protein, iron, antioxidants)
- 2 slices whole-grain toast (fiber)
- ½ cup sliced strawberries (antioxidants, fiber, potassium)

Lunch
- 2 cups grilled shrimp (4) and quinoa bowl with mixed vegetables (fiber, protein, magnesium, B vitamins)

Snack
- 1 small cucumber, sliced with 2 tablespoons tzatziki sauce (monounsaturated fats, potassium)

Dinner
- 6 ounces baked trout with a lemon-herb sauce (protein, omega-3s, vitamin D)
- 1 cup roasted Brussels sprouts (fiber, iron, potassium)
- 1 cup cooked brown rice (fiber, magnesium, vitamin B_6)

DAY 16

Breakfast
- 8 ounces Greek yogurt with 1 teaspoon honey and sliced peaches (antioxidants, calcium, vitamin B_{12})
- 20 almonds (monounsaturated fats, magnesium)

Lunch
- 2 cups chickpea and vegetable stir-fry (iron, magnesium, fiber, potassium)
- 1 cup mixed greens salad (antioxidants, fiber)

Snack
- 1 apple, sliced, with 1 tablespoon almond butter (monounsaturated fats, fiber)

Dinner
- 6 ounces grilled tilapia (protein, vitamin D)
- 1 cup steamed Swiss chard (calcium, potassium)
- ½ cup cooked quinoa (fiber, magnesium, vitamin B_6, vitamin B_9, vitamin B_{12})

DAY 17

Breakfast
- 12-ounce smoothie with kale, banana, chia seeds, and fortified almond milk (antioxidants, calcium, fiber, iron, magnesium, omega-3s, vitamin D), with optional ¼ cup whole-grain granola (protein, iron, vitamin D)

Lunch
- Turkey and avocado wrap with mixed greens in a whole-grain tortilla (protein, monounsaturated fats, fiber, antioxidants, magnesium)

Snack
- 1 cup carrot and celery sticks with 2 tablespoons hummus (monounsaturated fats, iron, antioxidants, calcium, potassium)

Dinner
- 6 ounces grilled swordfish with mango salsa (omega-3s, protein)

- 1 cup sautéed spinach (antioxidants, fiber, calcium, iron, magnesium, potassium)
- 1 cup cooked brown rice (fiber, magnesium, vitamin B$_6$)

DAY 18

Breakfast
- 2 scrambled eggs with spinach and feta cheese (antioxidants, fiber, calcium, iron, magnesium, potassium, protein)
- 1 slice whole-grain toast (fiber)
- 1 orange, sliced (vitamin C, antioxidants)

Lunch
- 2 cups quinoa salad with roasted vegetables and balsamic vinaigrette (fiber, magnesium, antioxidants)
- 1 cup mixed greens (calcium, fiber, iron)

Snack
- 1 cup sliced bell peppers and cucumber with 2 tablespoons hummus (monounsaturated fats, potassium)

Dinner
- 6 ounces grilled or baked salmon with a garlic-herb sauce (omega-3s, protein, vitamin D)
- 1 cup steamed broccoli (calcium, fiber, iron, magnesium)
- 1 cup cooked brown rice (fiber, magnesium, vitamin B$_6$)

DAY 19

Breakfast
- 1½ cups overnight oats with sliced strawberries and 1 tablespoon almond butter (antioxidants, fiber, potassium, monounsaturated fats) with 1 tablespoon chia seeds (antioxidants, calcium, fiber, iron, magnesium, omega-3s)

Lunch
- 2 cups lentil and vegetable stir-fry (iron, magnesium, potassium)
- 1 cup spinach and kale salad (antioxidants, fiber, calcium, iron, magnesium, potassium)

Snack
- ½ cup mixed nuts (fiber, monounsaturated fats, magnesium, protein)

Dinner
- 6-ounce grilled boneless, skinless chicken breast with a lemon-herb marinade (protein, vitamin B_{12})
- 1 cup sautéed spinach (antioxidants, fiber, calcium, iron, magnesium, potassium)
- ½ cup cooked quinoa (fiber, magnesium, vitamin B_6, vitamin B_9, vitamin B_{12})

DAY 20

Breakfast
- 12-ounce green smoothie with kale, pineapple, flaxseeds, and fortified almond milk (antioxidants, calcium, fiber, iron, magnesium, omega-3s, vitamin D) with ¼ cup whole-grain granola (protein, iron, vitamin D)

Lunch
- 2 cups turkey and avocado salad with mixed greens (protein, monounsaturated fats, antioxidants, fiber, magnesium)
- 1 whole-grain pita (fiber, iron, magnesium)

Snack
- 1 pear, sliced, with 1 tablespoon almond butter (monounsaturated fats, fiber)

Dinner
- 6 ounces baked cod with a lemon-dill sauce (omega-3s, vitamin D)
- 1 cup roasted asparagus (iron, potassium)
- 1 cup cooked brown rice (fiber, magnesium, vitamin B_6)

DAY 21

Breakfast
- 2 scrambled eggs with sautéed spinach and tomatoes (antioxidants, fiber, calcium, iron, magnesium, potassium, protein, vitamin B_{12})

- 1 slice whole-grain toast (fiber)
- 1 kiwi, sliced (vitamin C, antioxidants)

Lunch
- 2 cups quinoa and black bean salad with a lime vinaigrette (fiber, iron, magnesium)
- 1 cup mixed greens (calcium, fiber, antioxidants)

Snack
- 1 small cucumber, sliced, with 2 tablespoons tzatziki sauce (mono-unsaturated fats, potassium)

Dinner
- 6 ounces baked trout with a lemon-herb sauce (protein, omega-3s, vitamin D)
- 1 cup roasted Brussels sprouts (fiber, iron, potassium)
- 1 cup cooked brown rice (fiber, magnesium, vitamin B_6)

DAY 22

Breakfast
- 8 ounces Greek yogurt with 1 teaspoon honey and sliced peaches (antioxidants, calcium, vitamin B_{12})
- 20 almonds (monounsaturated fats, magnesium)

Lunch
- 2 cups chickpea and vegetable stir-fry (iron, magnesium, fiber, potassium)
- 1 cup spinach and kale salad (antioxidants, fiber, calcium, iron, magnesium, potassium)

Snack
- 1 apple, sliced, with 1 tablespoon almond butter (monounsaturated fats, fiber)

Dinner
- 6 ounces grilled swordfish with mango salsa (omega-3s, protein)

- 1 cup sautéed spinach (antioxidants, fiber, calcium, iron, magnesium, potassium)
- ½ cup cooked quinoa (fiber, magnesium, vitamin B_6, vitamin B_9, vitamin B_{12})

DAY 23

Breakfast
- 12-ounce smoothie with kale, banana, chia seeds, and fortified almond milk (antioxidants, calcium, fiber, iron, magnesium, omega-3s, vitamin D) with ¼ cup whole-grain granola (protein, iron, vitamin D)

Lunch
- Turkey and avocado wrap with mixed greens in a whole-grain tortilla (protein, monounsaturated fats, fiber, antioxidants, magnesium)

Snack
- 1 cup carrot and celery sticks with 2 tablespoons hummus (monounsaturated fats, calcium, iron, potassium)

Dinner
- 6 ounces grilled salmon with a lemon-dill sauce (omega-3s, protein, vitamin D)
- 1 cup steamed broccoli (calcium, fiber, iron, magnesium)
- 1 cup cooked brown rice (fiber, magnesium, vitamin B_6)

DAY 24

Breakfast
- 2 scrambled eggs with sautéed mushrooms and spinach (antioxidants, fiber, calcium, iron, magnesium, potassium, protein, vitamin B_{12})
- 1 slice whole-grain toast (fiber)
- 1 cup strawberries (antioxidants, fiber, potassium)

Lunch
- 2 cups quinoa and vegetable stir-fry with tofu (fiber, iron, magnesium, protein)
- 1 cup mixed greens (calcium, fiber, antioxidants)

Snack
- 1 cup sliced bell peppers and cucumber with 2 tablespoons hummus (antioxidants, monounsaturated fats, potassium)

Dinner
- 6 ounces baked cod with a lemon-herb sauce (omega-3s, protein, vitamin D)
- 1 cup roasted asparagus (iron, potassium)
- 1 cup cooked brown rice (fiber, magnesium, slow-burning carbs, vitamin B_6)

DAY 25

Breakfast
- 8 ounces Greek yogurt with 1 teaspoon honey and mixed berries (antioxidants, calcium, vitamin B_{12})
- 20 almonds (monounsaturated fats, magnesium)

Lunch
- 2 cups chickpea and vegetable salad with a tahini dressing (fiber, iron, magnesium, protein)
- 1 cup spinach and kale salad (antioxidants, fiber, calcium, iron, magnesium, potassium)

Snack
- 1 apple, sliced, with 1 tablespoon almond butter (monounsaturated fats, fiber)

Dinner
- 6 ounces grilled swordfish with mango salsa (omega-3s, protein)
- 1 cup sautéed spinach (antioxidants, fiber, calcium, iron, magnesium, potassium)
- ½ cup cooked quinoa (fiber, magnesium, vitamin B_6, vitamin B_9, vitamin B_{12})

DAY 26

Breakfast
- 12-ounce smoothie with kale, pineapple, chia seeds, and fortified almond milk (antioxidants, calcium, fiber, iron, magnesium, omega-3s, vitamin D) with ¼ cup whole-grain granola (protein, iron, vitamin D)

Lunch
- Turkey and avocado wrap with mixed greens in a whole-grain tortilla (protein, monounsaturated fats, fiber, antioxidants, magnesium)

Snack
- 1 cup carrot and celery sticks with 2 tablespoons hummus (monounsaturated fats, iron, calcium, potassium)

Dinner
- 6 ounces grilled salmon with a lemon-dill sauce (omega-3s, protein, vitamin D)
- 1 cup steamed broccoli (calcium, fiber, iron, magnesium)
- 1 cup cooked brown rice (fiber, magnesium, vitamin B_6)

DAY 27

Breakfast
- 2 scrambled eggs with sautéed spinach and tomatoes (antioxidants, fiber, calcium, iron, magnesium, potassium, protein, vitamin B_{12})
- 1 slice whole-grain toast (fiber)
- 1 sliced kiwi (vitamin C, antioxidants)

Lunch
- 2 cups quinoa and black bean salad with a lime vinaigrette (fiber, iron, protein, magnesium)
- 1 cup mixed greens (calcium, fiber, antioxidants)

Snack
- 1 small cucumber, sliced with 2 tablespoons tzatziki sauce (monounsaturated fats, potassium)

Dinner
- 6 ounces baked trout with a lemon-herb sauce (protein, omega-3s, vitamin D)
- 1 cup roasted Brussels sprouts (fiber, iron, potassium)
- 1 cup cooked brown rice (fiber, magnesium, vitamin B$_6$)

DAY 28

Breakfast
- 2 scrambled eggs with sautéed mushrooms and spinach (antioxidants, fiber, calcium, iron, magnesium, potassium, protein, vitamin B$_{12}$)
- 1 slice whole-grain toast (fiber)
- 1 cup strawberries (antioxidants, fiber, potassium)

Lunch
- 2 cups quinoa and black bean salad with a lime vinaigrette (fiber, iron, magnesium)
- 1 cup mixed greens (calcium, fiber, antioxidants)

Snack
- 1 small cucumber, sliced, with 2 tablespoons tzatziki sauce (monounsaturated fats, potassium)

Dinner
- 6 ounces baked trout with a lemon-herb sauce (protein, omega-3s, vitamin D)
- 1 cup roasted Brussels sprouts (fiber, iron, potassium)
- 1 cup cooked brown rice (fiber, magnesium, vitamin B$_6$)

DAY 29

Breakfast
- 8 ounces Greek yogurt with honey and mixed berries (antioxidants, calcium, vitamin B$_{12}$)
- 20 almonds (monounsaturated fats, magnesium)

Lunch
- 2 cups chickpea and vegetable stir-fry with tofu (iron, magnesium, protein)

- 1 cup spinach and kale salad (antioxidants, fiber, calcium, iron, magnesium, potassium, protein, vitamin B_{12})

Snack
- 1 apple, sliced, with 1 tablespoon almond butter (monounsaturated fats, fiber)

Dinner
- 6 ounces grilled swordfish with mango salsa (omega-3s, protein)
- 1 cup sautéed spinach (antioxidants, fiber, calcium, iron, magnesium, potassium)
- ½ cup cooked quinoa (fiber, magnesium, vitamin B_6, vitamin B_9, vitamin B_{12})

DAY 30

Breakfast
- 12-ounce smoothie with kale, pineapple, chia seeds, and fortified almond milk (antioxidants, calcium, fiber, iron, potassium, protein, omega-3s, vitamin D) with ¼ cup whole-grain granola (protein, iron, vitamin D)

Lunch
- Turkey and avocado wrap with mixed greens in a whole-grain tortilla (protein, monounsaturated fats, fiber, antioxidants, magnesium)

Snack
- 1 cup carrot and celery sticks with 2 tablespoons hummus (monounsaturated fats, iron, calcium, potassium)

Dinner
- 6 ounces grilled salmon with a lemon-dill sauce (omega-3s, protein, vitamin D)
- 1 cup steamed broccoli (calcium, fiber, iron, magnesium)
- 1 cup cooked brown rice (fiber, magnesium, vitamin B_6)

THE 50s

This is that proverbial pivotal decade that can decide the fate of the rest of your life. How you have treated your body in the past has been important, but this decade it really matters. All kinds of diseases pop up during these ten years, whether it's heart disease, high blood pressure, high cholesterol, or muscle loss. Nutrition can play a big role in preventing or treating many of these medical conditions. Antioxidants are a priority to help you fight disease at a microscopic level. Your vitamin intake is crucial, especially vitamin C to boost your immunity, and vitamin D to protect your bones and heart. Getting enough high-fiber foods is important to keep your gastrointestinal tract regular. Food should always be fun, but in this decade more than any other, food can also be thought of as medicinal to not only heal but protect your body.

BREAKFAST

- 8-ounce Greek yogurt parfait with berries (antioxidants, calcium, protein) and chia seeds (fiber, omega-3s)
- 1 cup cooked oatmeal topped with strawberries and flaxseeds (fiber, antioxidants, vitamin B_9), 2 scrambled eggs (protein, vitamin B_{12})
- 2 hard-boiled eggs (protein, vitamin B_{12}), 1 slice whole-grain toast with almond butter (fiber, monounsaturated fats), ½ cup blueberries (antioxidants, fiber)
- 8 ounces Greek yogurt with honey and mixed berries (antioxidants, calcium, protein) and walnuts (monounsaturated fats, omega-3s)
- 2 small whole-grain pancakes with sliced bananas and 1 tablespoon almond butter (fiber, monounsaturated fats), 1 cup orange juice (vitamin C)
- 8-ounce smoothie made with milk or juice, kale, banana, and

chia seeds (fiber, vitamin C), 1 hard-boiled egg (protein, vitamin B_{12})

- 1 cup cottage cheese and sliced peaches (protein, calcium, vitamin C), 1 slice whole-grain toast with almond butter (fiber, monounsaturated fats)
- 2 small whole-grain pancakes with blueberry compote (fiber, antioxidants, vitamin B_9), ½ cup Greek yogurt (calcium, protein)
- 1½ cups cooked oatmeal with sliced banana and ¼ cup walnuts (fiber, monounsaturated fats, vitamin B_9), 1 scrambled egg (protein, vitamin B_{12})
- 2-egg spinach and cheddar cheese–stuffed omelet (protein, calcium), 1 slice whole-grain toast with almond butter (fiber, monounsaturated fats), 1 cup freshly squeezed grapefruit juice (vitamin C)
- 1½ cups overnight oats with sliced peaches and ¼ cup chopped pecans (fiber, monounsaturated fats, vitamin B_9), 1 scrambled egg (protein, vitamin B_{12})
- 2 small whole-grain waffles with almond butter and sliced bananas (fiber, monounsaturated fats), 1 cup freshly squeezed orange juice (vitamin C)
- 2 cups açai bowl with mixed berries, granola, and a drizzle of honey (antioxidants, fiber)
- 1 cup cottage cheese with sliced peaches and a sprinkle of flaxseeds (calcium, fiber)
- 3 ounces smoked salmon and 1 tablespoon cream cheese on both halves of a whole-grain bagel with capers and red onion (protein, omega-3s, vitamin B_{12})
- 12-ounce smoothie with kale, banana, and almond milk (fiber, antioxidants, vitamin B_9)
- 1½ cups oatmeal with sliced strawberries and a sprinkle of chia seeds (fiber, vitamin B_9)
- 8 ounces Greek yogurt with berries and a sprinkle of flaxseeds (antioxidants, calcium, fiber, protein)

- 12-ounce smoothie with milk or juice, spinach, blueberries, and a scoop of protein powder (antioxidants, protein)
- 1 cup cottage cheese with mixed berries and a drizzle of honey (calcium, antioxidants)
- 1 slice whole-wheat toast with avocado and a poached egg (monounsaturated fats, protein)
- 12-ounce almond milk smoothie with spinach, kiwi, and a scoop of protein powder (antioxidants, protein)

LUNCH

- Spinach and kale salad with 3 ounces grilled boneless, skinless chicken breast, diced (fiber, protein, vitamin C), ½ small avocado, sliced (monounsaturated fats), and ¼ cup almonds (vitamin E, monounsaturated fats)
- 2 cups quinoa and black bean salad with avocado (fiber, monounsaturated fats) and sliced oranges (vitamin C)
- 1 cup lentil soup (fiber, protein), small spinach and tomato salad (vitamin C)
- 1½ cups tuna salad, mixed greens (protein, omega-3s) with sliced strawberries (vitamin C)
- Turkey and avocado wrap on whole-grain tortilla (fiber, monounsaturated fats), ½ cup mixed berries (antioxidants, fiber)
- ½ cup chickpea and ½ cup spinach (cooked) curry (fiber, protein), 1 cup cooked brown rice (fiber)
- 3 cups quinoa and mixed veggie salad with feta cheese (fiber, calcium) and kiwi slices (vitamin C)
- 3 cups quinoa and chickpea salad with mixed vegetables (fiber, protein) and kiwi slices (vitamin C)
- 2 cups lentil and vegetable stir-fry (fiber, protein) with orange sections (vitamin C)
- Turkey and cranberry sandwich on 2 slices whole-grain bread with ½ cup mixed berries (antioxidants, fiber, protein)

- 3 cups chickpea and spinach salad with feta cheese (fiber, protein, calcium) and sliced mango (vitamin C)
- 3 cups spinach and walnut salad with grilled boneless, skinless chicken breast (fiber, protein) and sliced strawberries (vitamin C)
- 2 cups quinoa and black bean burrito bowl (fiber, protein) with kiwi slices (vitamin C)
- 3 cups spinach and kale salad with grilled shrimp (4) (fiber, protein) and avocado slices (monounsaturated fats), and ¼ cup halved almonds (vitamin E, monounsaturated fats)
- 1½ cups lentil and vegetable soup (fiber, protein), 1 kiwi (vitamin C), or 1 cup of melon such as cantaloupe (vitamin C)
- Turkey and avocado wrap on whole-grain tortilla (fiber, monounsaturated fats), 1 orange (vitamin C)
- 3 cups quinoa salad with roasted vegetables, 3 sliced strawberries, and feta cheese (fiber, protein, calcium, vitamin C)
- 2 cups shrimp (6) and avocado salad with mixed greens and a balsamic vinaigrette (protein, monounsaturated fats, vitamin B_{12})
- 6-ounce spinach and mushroom–stuffed chicken breast with quinoa (protein, fiber)
- 2 cups black bean and corn salad with grilled boneless, skinless chicken breast and a lime-cilantro dressing (protein, fiber, vitamin C)
- 1½ cups lentil and vegetable soup with a side of mixed greens (fiber, vitamin B_9)
- 2 cups whole-wheat pasta salad with tomatoes, spinach, and extra-virgin olive oil (fiber, monounsaturated fats)
- 3 cups spinach and chickpea salad with a lemon-tahini dressing (fiber, vitamin C)
- 2 cups whole-wheat pasta with a tomato and vegetable sauce (fiber, vitamin C)
- 3 cups spinach and walnut salad with a vinaigrette dressing (antioxidants, monounsaturated fats)
- 2 cups quinoa and black bean salad with a lime-cilantro dressing (fiber, vitamin C)

- 2 cups whole-wheat pasta with pesto sauce and cherry tomatoes (monounsaturated fats, vitamin C)

DINNER

- 6 ounces baked salmon (omega-3s, protein, vitamin D) with steamed broccoli (fiber, vitamin C) and ½ cup cooked quinoa (protein, fiber)
- 4 to 6 grilled shrimp (protein), 4 asparagus spears (fiber, vitamin D), ½ cup brown rice (fiber)
- 6-ounce baked boneless, skinless chicken breast with lemon and rosemary (protein, vitamin C), 1 cup cooked steamed kale (fiber, calcium), ½ cup cooked quinoa (protein, vitamin B$_9$)
- 6 ounces grilled salmon (protein, omega-3s), ½ cup roasted Brussels sprouts (fiber, vitamin C), 1 cup diced roasted sweet potatoes (fiber, vitamin A)
- 6 ounces baked cod with a side of spinach (protein, calcium, vitamin D), ½ cup cooked quinoa (protein, fiber)
- 6 ounces grilled tofu with broccoli (protein, calcium, fiber), 1 cup mashed sweet potatoes (fiber, vitamin A)
- 6-ounce baked or grilled boneless, skinless chicken breast with roasted cauliflower (protein, fiber, vitamin C), 1 cup brown rice (fiber)
- 6 ounces baked or grilled trout (omega-3s, protein), 1 cup steamed broccoli (fiber, vitamin C), ½ cup mashed sweet potatoes (fiber, vitamin A)
- 6 ounces grilled chicken with a side of asparagus (protein, fiber), 1 cup quinoa (protein, vitamin B$_9$)
- 6 ounces baked cod with a side of spinach (protein, calcium, vitamin D), ½ cup brown rice (fiber)
- 6 grilled shrimp skewers with zucchini (protein)
- 6 ounces baked tofu with roasted Brussels sprouts (protein, fiber) and ½ cup quinoa (protein, vitamin B$_9$)
- 6-ounce baked or grilled pork chop with lemon and rosemary

(protein, vitamin C), 1 cup steamed broccoli (fiber, vitamin D), ½ cup brown rice (fiber)

- 6 ounces grilled or baked tilapia with a side of steamed kale (protein, calcium, vitamin D), ½ cup cooked quinoa (protein, fiber) or brown rice (protein, fiber)
- 6 ounces grilled swordfish with a mango salsa (omega-3s, protein), 1 cup roasted Brussels sprouts (fiber, vitamin C), ½ cup cooked quinoa (protein, vitamin B_9)
- 6-ounce steak (protein, iron) or grilled boneless, skinless chicken breast with lemon and thyme (protein, vitamin C), 1 cup steamed broccoli (fiber, vitamin D), ½ cup cooked brown rice (fiber)
- 6 ounces grilled or baked salmon with a dill and yogurt sauce (omega-3s, protein), 4 asparagus spears (fiber, vitamin D), ½ cup mashed sweet potatoes (fiber, vitamin A)
- 6 ounces baked cod with a lemon-herb crust (protein, omega-3s), 1 cup cooked quinoa (protein, vitamin B_9)
- 6 ounces grilled tuna or swordfish with ½ cup cooked quinoa and 4 medium roasted asparagus spears (protein, omega-3s)
- 6 ounces baked sea bass or cod with 1 small baked sweet potato and ½ cup sautéed spinach (protein, fiber, vitamin B_9)
- 6 ounces baked or grilled trout or tilapia with 1 cup brown rice and ½ cup steamed broccoli (protein, fiber)
- 6 ounces grilled mackerel with 1 cup wild rice and 1 cup sautéed Brussels sprouts (omega-3s, fiber, vitamin D)
- 6 ounces grilled trout with 1 cup wild rice and ½ cup steamed broccoli (omega-3s, fiber, vitamin D)
- 6-ounce grilled boneless, skinless chicken breast with ½ cup quinoa and 4 medium sautéed asparagus spears (protein, fiber)
- 6 ounces grilled salmon with ½ cup steamed broccoli and ½ cup quinoa (omega-3s, protein, vitamin D)
- 6 ounces grilled tofu with ½ cup sautéed kale and ½ cup quinoa (protein, vitamin B_{12})
- 6 grilled shrimp with 1 cup quinoa and 4 sautéed asparagus spears (protein, omega-3s)

- 6 ounces grilled chicken with a side of 1 cup diced roasted butternut squash and ½ cup broccoli (protein, vitamin B$_9$)
- 6 ounces grilled or baked salmon with a side of ½ cup quinoa and ½ cup steamed green beans (omega-3s, protein)

SNACKS

- ½ cup Greek yogurt with ¼ cup mixed berries and 1 tablespoon almonds (antioxidants, calcium, protein, monounsaturated fats)
- 2 ounces smoked salmon on whole-grain crackers with small avocado slices (omega 3s, protein, fiber, monounsaturated fats, vitamin C)
- ¼ avocado on 2 whole-grain crackers (omega-3s, protein, monounsaturated fats)
- 1 cup edamame beans (protein, fiber, calcium, vitamin C)
- 1 cup baby carrots and ½ bell pepper, sliced, with 2 tablespoons hummus (fiber, vitamin C, protein, monounsaturated fats)
- 2 hard-boiled eggs and ½ cup grape tomatoes (protein, vitamin B$_{12}$, vitamin D, antioxidants)
- ½ cup cottage cheese with 1 small peach, sliced, and 1 tablespoon chia seeds (calcium, protein, fiber)
- ¼ cup mixed nuts with 2 tablespoons dried cranberries (fiber, monounsaturated fats, omega-3s, protein, antioxidants)
- 3 ounces canned tuna with 1 cup mixed greens and ½ cup cherry tomatoes (omega-3s, protein, vitamin B$_{12}$, vitamin C)
- 1 medium apple, sliced, with 1 tablespoon almond butter (fiber, monounsaturated fats)
- 12-ounce smoothie made with 1 cup spinach, 1 medium banana, 1 cup almond milk, 1 tablespoon chia seeds, 1 scoop protein powder (vitamin B$_9$, vitamin C, calcium, protein, omega-3s)
- 1 slice whole-grain bread with ¼ avocado (fiber, monounsaturated fats, vitamin C, omega-3s, protein)
- 1 large tomato, sliced (vitamin C)
- 1 cup carrot and cucumber sticks (fiber, antioxidants)

- 1 cup bell pepper, sliced (vitamin C)
- ¼ cup mixed nuts, such as almonds and walnuts, with ¼ cup dried fruit (antioxidants, fiber, magnesium, monounsaturated fats, protein)
- ½ cup cooked quinoa with diced cucumber and tomato, 1 tablespoon chopped walnuts, fresh parsley (protein, fiber, antioxidants, vitamin C, monounsaturated fats, omega-3s, vitamin B$_9$)
- ½ cup roasted chickpeas seasoned with paprika, garlic powder, and a pinch of salt, with tzatziki sauce (protein, fiber)

Now that you have some examples of the types of meals and snacks you can eat and the power nutrients they contain, you can mix and match them to create daily meal plans. Below you will find menus with approximately 2,000 to 2,500 calories per day, but if you want to eat less, you can make adjustments to bring this calorie count lower. This is meant to be a stress-free, flexible plan that you will enjoy. You can make reasonable substitutions such as swapping brown rice for quinoa and vice versa. You can mix days by taking meals or snacks from one day and substituting it in another day. For example, if you don't have the ingredients for dinner on day 2, but you have the ingredients for dinner on day 7, then you can have the day 7 dinner on day 2. The idea is to get as much of your top 10 food nutrients into your diet as possible and have fun while doing it.

30-DAY MEAL PLAN

DAY 1

Breakfast
- 8-ounce Greek yogurt parfait with berries (antioxidants, calcium, protein), 1 tablespoon chia seeds (fiber, omega-3s)

Lunch
- 3 cups spinach and kale salad with 3-ounce grilled boneless, skinless chicken breast, diced (fiber, protein, vitamin C), ½ small avocado, sliced (monounsaturated fats), and almonds (vitamin E, monounsaturated fats)

Snack

- 1 small carrot, sliced, or 1 small cucumber, sliced, with 2 tablespoons hummus (fiber, vitamin C)

Dinner

- 6 ounces baked salmon (omega-3s, protein, vitamin D) with 1 cup steamed broccoli (fiber, vitamin C) and ½ cup cooked quinoa (protein, fiber)

Snack

- ½ cup Greek yogurt with a drizzle of honey (calcium, protein, vitamin B_{12})

DAY 2

Breakfast

- 1 cup cooked oatmeal topped with strawberries and ½ tablespoon flaxseeds (fiber, antioxidants, vitamin B_9)
- 2 scrambled eggs (protein, vitamin B_{12})

Lunch

- 2 cups quinoa and black bean salad with ½ small avocado, sliced (fiber, monounsaturated fats), and orange sections from 1 medium orange (vitamin C)

Snack

- 20 mixed nuts (fiber, monounsaturated fats, magnesium, protein)

Dinner

- 4 to 6 grilled shrimp (protein)
- 4 asparagus spears (fiber, vitamin D)
- ½ cup brown rice (fiber)

DAY 3

Breakfast

- 1 slice whole-grain toast with 1 teaspoon almond butter (fiber, monounsaturated fats)
- ½ cup blueberries (antioxidants, fiber)
- 2 hard-boiled eggs (protein, vitamin B_{12})

Lunch
- 1 cup lentil soup (fiber, protein)
- 1 cup spinach and tomato salad (vitamin C)

Snack
- 1 small bell pepper, sliced, with 2 tablespoons guacamole (fiber, monounsaturated fats)

Dinner
- 6-ounce baked boneless, skinless chicken breast with lemon and rosemary (protein, vitamin C)
- 1 cup steamed kale (fiber, calcium)
- ½ cup cooked quinoa (protein, vitamin B_9)

DAY 4

Breakfast
- 8 ounces Greek yogurt with 1 teaspoon honey and ¼ cup mixed berries (antioxidants, calcium, protein) and walnuts (monounsaturated fats, omega-3s)

Lunch
- 1½ cups tuna salad with mixed greens (protein, omega-3s) and sliced strawberries (vitamin C)

Snack
- Edamame (protein, fiber, vitamin B_9)

Dinner
- 6 ounces grilled salmon (protein, omega-3s)
- ½ cup roasted Brussels sprouts (fiber, vitamin C)
- 1 cup diced roasted sweet potatoes (fiber, vitamin A)

DAY 5

Breakfast
- 2 small whole-grain pancakes with ¼ small banana, sliced, and 1 tablespoon almond butter (fiber, monounsaturated fats)
- 1 cup freshly squeezed orange juice (vitamin C)

Lunch
- Turkey and avocado wrap on a whole-grain tortilla (fiber, monounsaturated fats)
- ½ cup mixed berries (antioxidants, fiber)

Snack
- ½ cup cottage cheese (protein, calcium)
- ½ cup baby carrots (fiber, vitamin A)

Dinner
- 6 ounces baked cod with a side of ½ cup cooked spinach (protein, calcium, vitamin D)
- ½ cup cooked quinoa (protein, fiber)

DAY 6

Breakfast
- 8-ounce smoothie with kale, pineapple, and chia seeds (fiber, vitamin C)
- 1 hard-boiled egg (protein, vitamin B_{12})

Lunch
- ½ cup chickpea and 1 cup cooked spinach curry (fiber, protein)
- 2 cups brown rice (fiber)

Snack
- ½ cup almonds and dried cranberries (monounsaturated fats, antioxidants, fiber)

Dinner
- 6 ounces grilled tofu with ½ cup broccoli (protein, calcium, fiber)
- 1 cup mashed sweet potatoes (fiber, vitamin A)

DAY 7

Breakfast
- 1 cup cottage cheese and sliced peaches (protein, calcium, vitamin C)
- 1 slice whole-grain toast (fiber)

Lunch
- 3 cups quinoa salad with mixed veggies, ¼ cup feta cheese (fiber, calcium), and 1 kiwi, sliced (vitamin C)

Snack
- 6 celery sticks with 1 tablespoon peanut butter (fiber, monounsaturated fats)

Dinner
- 6-ounce baked or grilled boneless, skinless chicken breast with roasted cauliflower (protein, fiber, vitamin C)
- 1 cup brown rice (fiber)

DAY 8

Breakfast
- 2-egg spinach and mushroom omelet (protein, vitamin B_{12})
- 1 slice whole-grain toast with avocado (fiber, monounsaturated fats)
- 1 cup freshly squeezed orange juice (vitamin C)

Lunch
- 3 cups quinoa and chickpea salad with mixed vegetables (fiber, protein) and 1 kiwi, sliced (vitamin C)

Snack
- ½ cup mixed nuts and dried apricots (protein, magnesium, monounsaturated fats, fiber)

Dinner
- 6 ounces baked or grilled trout (omega-3s, protein)
- 1 cup steamed broccoli (fiber, vitamin C)
- ½ cup mashed sweet potatoes (fiber, vitamin A)

DAY 9

Breakfast
- 8-ounce Greek yogurt parfait with pomegranate seeds (antioxidants, calcium, protein) and flaxseed sprinkles (fiber, omega-3s)

Lunch
- 2 cups lentil and vegetable stir-fry (fiber, protein) with 1 orange (vitamin C)

Snack
- 1 small red bell pepper, sliced, with 2 tablespoons hummus (fiber, monounsaturated fats)

Dinner
- 6-ounce grilled boneless, skinless chicken breast with a side of 4 medium asparagus spears (protein, fiber)
- 1 cup quinoa (protein, vitamin B_9)

DAY 10

Breakfast
- 2 small whole-grain waffles with 1 cup strawberries and a drizzle of honey (fiber, antioxidants, vitamin B_9)
- 1 scrambled egg (protein, vitamin B_{12})

Lunch
- Turkey and cranberry sandwich on 2 slices whole-grain bread (fiber, protein)
- ½ cup mixed berries (antioxidants, fiber)

Snack
- ½ cup cottage cheese with pineapple chunks (protein, calcium, vitamin C)

Dinner
- 6 ounces baked cod with a side of ½ cup spinach, cooked (protein, calcium, vitamin D)
- ½ cup brown rice (fiber)

DAY 11

Breakfast
- 8-ounce smoothie with milk or juice, kale, banana, and chia seeds (fiber, vitamin C)
- 1 hard-boiled egg (protein, vitamin B_{12})

Lunch
- 3 cups chickpea and spinach salad with ¼ cup feta cheese (fiber, protein, calcium) and 2 mango slices (vitamin C)

Snack
- ½ cup almonds and dried blueberries (monounsaturated fats, antioxidants, fiber)

Dinner
- 6 grilled shrimp skewers with ½ cup diced roasted zucchini (protein)
- ½ cup quinoa or brown rice (protein, fiber)

DAY 12

Breakfast
- 1 cup cottage cheese and sliced peaches (protein, calcium, vitamin C)
- 1 slice whole-grain toast with 1 teaspoon almond butter (fiber, monounsaturated fats)

Lunch
- 3 cups spinach and walnut salad with grilled boneless, skinless chicken breast (fiber, protein) and 1 cup strawberries, sliced (vitamin C)

Snack
- 6 carrot sticks with 2 tablespoons guacamole (fiber, monounsaturated fats)

Dinner
- 6 ounces baked tofu with 1 cup roasted Brussels sprouts (protein, fiber)
- ½ cup quinoa (protein, vitamin B_9)

DAY 13

Breakfast
- 2 small whole-grain pancakes with blueberry compote (fiber, antioxidants, vitamin B_9)
- ½ cup Greek yogurt (calcium, protein)

Lunch

- 2 cups quinoa and black bean burrito bowl (fiber, protein) with 1 kiwi, sliced (vitamin C)

Snack

- ½ cup mixed nuts and dried cranberries (magnesium, monounsaturated fats, antioxidants, fiber)

Dinner

- 6-ounce baked or grilled pork chop with lemon and rosemary (protein, vitamin C)
- 1 cup steamed broccoli (fiber, vitamin D)
- ½ cup brown rice (fiber)

DAY 14

Breakfast

- 1½ cups cooked oatmeal with ¼ small banana, sliced, and ¼ cup walnuts (fiber, monounsaturated fats, vitamin B_9)
- 1 scrambled egg (protein, vitamin B_{12})

Lunch

- 3 cups spinach and kale salad with 4 grilled shrimp (fiber, protein) and ½ small avocado, sliced (monounsaturated fats), and ¼ cup halved almonds (vitamin E, monounsaturated fats)

Snack

- ½ medium cucumber, sliced, with 2 tablespoons hummus (fiber, vitamin C)

Dinner

- 6 ounces grilled or baked tilapia with a side of ½ cup steamed kale (protein, calcium, vitamin D)
- ½ cup cooked quinoa or brown rice (protein, fiber)

DAY 15

Breakfast

- 2-egg spinach and cheddar cheese–stuffed omelet (protein, calcium)

- 1 slice whole-grain toast with 1 teaspoon almond butter (fiber, monounsaturated fats)
- 1 cup freshly squeezed grapefruit juice (vitamin C)

Lunch
- 1½ cups lentil and vegetable soup (fiber, protein)
- 1 kiwi, sliced (vitamin C), or 1 cup melon such as cantaloupe (vitamin C)

Snack
- ½ cup Greek yogurt with 1 cup mixed berries (antioxidants, calcium, protein)

Dinner
- 6 ounces grilled swordfish with a mango salsa (omega-3s, protein)
- 1 cup roasted Brussels sprouts (fiber, vitamin C)
- ½ cup cooked quinoa (protein, vitamin B$_9$)

DAY 16

Breakfast
- 1½ cups overnight oats with ¼ cup sliced peaches and ½ cup chopped pecans (fiber, monounsaturated fats, vitamin B$_9$)
- 1 scrambled egg (protein, vitamin B$_{12}$)

Lunch
- Turkey and avocado wrap on a whole-grain tortilla (fiber, monounsaturated fats)
- 1 orange (vitamin C)

Snack
- 6 carrot sticks with 2 tablespoons tzatziki dip (fiber, vitamin A)

Dinner
- 6-ounce steak (protein, iron) or grilled boneless, skinless chicken breast with lemon and thyme (protein, vitamin C)
- 1 cup steamed broccoli (fiber, vitamin D)
- ½ cup cooked brown rice (fiber)

DAY 17

Breakfast
- 8-ounce Greek yogurt parfait with mixed berries and honey (antioxidants, calcium, protein) and 1 tablespoon chia seeds (fiber, omega-3s)

Lunch
- 3 cups quinoa salad with roasted vegetables and feta cheese (fiber, protein, calcium) and sliced strawberries (vitamin C)

Snack
- ½ cup mixed nuts and dried apricots (magnesium, monounsaturated fats, fiber, protein)

Dinner
- 6 ounces grilled or baked salmon with a dill and yogurt sauce (omega-3s, protein)
- 4 asparagus spears (fiber, vitamin D)
- ½ cup mashed sweet potatoes (fiber, vitamin A)

DAY 18

Breakfast
- 2 small or 1 large whole-grain waffle with 1 tablespoon almond butter and sliced bananas (fiber, monounsaturated fats)
- 1 cup freshly squeezed orange juice (vitamin C)

Lunch
- 2 cups chickpea and spinach curry (fiber, protein) with 2 mango slices (vitamin C)

Snack
- 1 bell pepper, sliced, with 2 tablespoons hummus (fiber, monounsaturated fats)

Dinner
- 6 ounces baked cod with a lemon-herb crust (protein, omega-3s)
- 1 cup cooked quinoa (protein, vitamin B_9)

DAY 19

Breakfast
- 2 cups açai bowl with mixed berries, 1 tablespoon granola, and a drizzle of honey (antioxidants, fiber)

Snack
- 1 mango, sliced (vitamin C)

Lunch
- 6 shrimp on a bed of salad made with ½ small avocado, sliced, and 2 cups mixed greens and a balsamic vinaigrette (protein, monounsaturated fats, vitamin B_{12})

Snack
- ½ cup mixed nuts and dried cherries (magnesium, monounsaturated fats, fiber, protein, antioxidants)

Dinner
- 6 ounces grilled tuna or swordfish with ½ cup quinoa and 4 medium roasted asparagus spears (protein, omega-3s)

DAY 20

Breakfast
- 1 cup cottage cheese with sliced peaches and a sprinkle of flaxseed (calcium, fiber)

Snack
- 1 medium kiwi, sliced (vitamin C)

Lunch
- 6-ounce spinach and mushroom–stuffed chicken breast with ½ cup quinoa (protein, fiber)

Snack
- 1 medium sliced cucumber with 2 tablespoons tzatziki sauce (fiber, vitamin C)

Dinner
- 6 ounces baked sea bass or cod with 1 small baked sweet potato and ½ cup sautéed spinach (protein, fiber, vitamin B_9)

DAY 21

Breakfast
- 3 ounces smoked salmon and 1 teaspoon cream cheese on both halves of a whole-grain bagel with capers and red onion (protein, omega-3s, vitamin B$_{12}$)

Snack
- 1 cup Greek yogurt with mixed berries (antioxidants, calcium, vitamin C)

Lunch
- 2 cups black bean and corn salad with grilled chicken and a lime-cilantro dressing (protein, fiber, vitamin C)

Snack
- 1 pear, sliced, with 1 tablespoon almond butter (monounsaturated fats, fiber, vitamin B$_9$)

Dinner
- 6 ounces baked or grilled trout or tilapia with ½ cup brown rice and ½ cup steamed broccoli (protein, fiber)

DAY 22

Breakfast
- 2 small whole-grain pancakes with fresh blueberries and a drizzle of maple syrup (fiber, antioxidants)

Snack
- 1 cup edamame (protein, antioxidants)

Lunch
- 2 cups quinoa and black bean bowl with ¼ cup guacamole and salsa (fiber, monounsaturated fats, vitamin B$_9$)

Snack
- ½ cup mixed nuts and dried apricots (fiber, magnesium, monounsaturated fats, protein, antioxidants)

Dinner
- 6 ounces grilled mackerel with ½ cup wild rice and 1 cup roasted Brussels sprouts (omega-3s, fiber, vitamin D)

DAY 23

Breakfast
- 12-ounce smoothie with kale, banana, and almond milk (fiber, antioxidants, vitamin B_9)

Snack
- ½ cup mixed nuts and dried cranberries (fiber, magnesium, monounsaturated fats, antioxidants, protein)

Lunch
- 1½ cups lentil and vegetable soup with a side of 1 cup mixed greens (fiber, protein, vitamin B_9)

Snack
- 1 cup carrot sticks and cucumber slices with 2 tablespoons hummus (fiber, antioxidants)

Dinner
- 6 ounces grilled trout with ½ cup wild rice and ½ cup steamed broccoli (protein, omega-3s, fiber, vitamin D)

DAY 24

Breakfast
- 1½ cups oatmeal with 1 cup strawberries, sliced, and 1 tablespoon chia seeds (fiber, vitamin B_9)

Snack
- 1 orange (vitamin C) with ½ cup walnuts (protein, omega 3, antioxidants, fiber)

Lunch
- 1½ cups chickpea and spinach curry with 1½ cups brown rice (protein, fiber, vitamin B_9)

Snack
- ½ cup mixed berries (antioxidants, vitamin C)

Dinner
- 6-ounce grilled boneless, skinless chicken breast with ½ cup quinoa and ½ cup sautéed asparagus (protein, fiber)

DAY 25

Breakfast
- 8 ounces Greek yogurt with berries and 1 teaspoon flaxseeds (antioxidants, calcium, fiber, protein)

Lunch
- 2 cups whole-wheat pasta salad with tomatoes, spinach, and extra-virgin olive oil (fiber, monounsaturated fats)

Dinner
- 6 ounces grilled salmon with ½ cup steamed broccoli and ½ cup quinoa (omega-3s, protein, vitamin D)

DAY 26

Breakfast
- 1½ cups oatmeal with 1 tablespoon almond butter and ½ small banana, sliced (fiber, monounsaturated fats)

Lunch
- 3 cups spinach and chickpea salad with a lemon-tahini dressing (fiber, vitamin C)

Dinner
- 6-ounce grilled or baked boneless, skinless chicken breast with 4 medium asparagus spears and ½ cup brown rice (protein, vitamin B_9)

DAY 27

Breakfast
- 12-ounce smoothie with milk or juice, spinach, blueberries, and a scoop of protein powder (antioxidants, protein)

Lunch
- 2 cups whole-wheat pasta with a tomato and vegetable sauce (fiber, vitamin C)

Dinner
- 6 ounces grilled tofu with ½ cup sautéed kale and ½ cup quinoa (protein, vitamin B_{12})

DAY 28

Breakfast
- 1 cup cottage cheese with mixed berries and a drizzle of honey (calcium, antioxidants)

Lunch
- 3 cups spinach and walnut salad with a vinaigrette dressing (antioxidants, monounsaturated fats)

Dinner
- 6 grilled shrimp with 1 cup quinoa and ½ cup sautéed asparagus (protein, omega-3s)

DAY 29

Breakfast
- 1 slice whole-wheat toast with ½ small avocado, sliced, and 1 poached egg (monounsaturated fats, protein)

Lunch
- 2 cups quinoa and black bean salad with a lime-cilantro dressing (fiber, vitamin C)

Dinner
- 6-ounce grilled boneless, skinless chicken breast with a side of 1 cup diced roasted butternut squash and ½ cup broccoli (protein, vitamin B_9)

DAY 30

Breakfast
- 12-ounce almond milk smoothie with spinach, kiwi, and a scoop of protein powder (antioxidants, protein)

Lunch
- 2 cups whole-wheat pasta with pesto sauce and cherry tomatoes (monounsaturated fats, vitamin C)

Dinner
- 6 ounces grilled or baked salmon with 1 cup quinoa and 1 cup steamed green beans (omega-3s, protein)

THE 60s+

As we age, we tend to eat less, and our bodies start shrinking, not just in stature but muscularity and flexibility. These decades after 60 are likely to see the most changes in our bodies and the greatest vulnerability to various diseases and medical conditions. While years of nutrition and exercise choices as well as genetics make us more vulnerable to illness unlike the other decades, all is far from lost. It is absolutely possible to live a robust, energetic, and pleasurable life in these years. Part of what will allow you to do that starts at the table. Consuming foods high in calcium, protein, fiber, and omega-3s remains critical and is important for brain and heart health. In this decade, it's important to eat not just to power your body but your mind as well.

BREAKFAST

- 8-ounce Greek yogurt parfait with berries (antioxidants, calcium, protein) and 1 tablespoon chia seeds (fiber, omega-3s)
- 1½ cups oatmeal topped with banana and walnuts (fiber, magnesium, potassium)

- 1 slice whole-grain toast with avocado and 2 poached eggs (fiber, vitamin D, vitamin B_{12})
- Spinach and feta 2-egg omelet (protein, calcium, vitamin B_6, vitamin B_{12})
- 12-ounce smoothie with spinach, banana, almond milk, and flaxseeds (fiber, potassium, vitamin B_6)
- 2 whole-grain pancakes with fresh blueberries (fiber, vitamin B_6, vitamin B_9)
- 1 cup cottage cheese and mixed fruit salad (calcium, vitamin B_{12})
- 2 scrambled eggs with sautéed spinach and whole-grain toast (protein, vitamin B_6, vitamin B_9)
- 2 small or 1 large whole-grain waffle with strawberries and a drizzle of maple syrup (fiber, vitamin B_6, vitamin B_9)
- 1½ cups overnight oats with almond butter, banana, and 1 tablespoon chia seeds (fiber, magnesium, potassium)
- 12-ounce smoothie with kale, pineapple, Greek yogurt, and flaxseeds (fiber, calcium, vitamin B_6)
- 1 slice avocado and smoked salmon toast (omega-3s, vitamin D, vitamin B_{12})
- 1 cup cottage cheese with sliced peaches and a sprinkle of almonds (calcium, vitamin B_{12})
- 1½ cups whole-grain cereal with almond milk and sliced strawberries (fiber, vitamin B_6, vitamin B_9)
- 8 ounces Greek yogurt with mixed berries and 1 tablespoon chia seeds (calcium, fiber, protein, omega-3s, vitamin B_6)
- 12-ounce smoothie with kale, banana, chia seeds, and almond milk (fiber, potassium, omega-3s)
- 2 cottage cheese pancakes with blueberries (calcium, protein, fiber)
- 2 small or 1 large whole-grain waffle with strawberries and a drizzle of honey (fiber, potassium)
- 1½ cups whole-grain cereal with low-fat milk (calcium, B_{12})
- 2 scrambled eggs with sautéed spinach and whole-grain toast (protein, fiber, B_6, B_9)

LUNCH

- 6 ounces grilled salmon with ½ cup quinoa and ½ cup steamed broccoli (protein, omega-3s, magnesium, fiber)
- 1½ cups lentil soup and a small spinach salad (protein, fiber, magnesium, vitamin B_6, vitamin B_9)
- 2 cups quinoa and black bean salad with a side of ¼ cup guacamole (protein, magnesium, vitamin B_6)
- 1 cup tuna salad with mixed greens and whole-grain crackers (omega-3s, vitamin D)
- 1½ cups chickpea and vegetable stir-fry with brown rice (protein, magnesium, vitamin B_6)
- Turkey and avocado wrap with a side of mixed greens (protein, vitamin B_9, magnesium)
- 3 cups spinach and kale salad with 3 ounces grilled chicken breast, diced (protein, vitamin B_6, vitamin B_9)
- 6 ounces grilled tilapia with ½ cup quinoa and 1 cup mixed greens salad (protein, omega-3s, magnesium)
- 2 cups black bean and corn salad with 3 grilled shrimp (protein, magnesium, vitamin B_6)
- 2 cups turkey and vegetable stir-fry with ½ cup brown rice (protein, magnesium, vitamin B_6)
- 2 cups lentil and vegetable curry with whole-grain naan bread (protein, magnesium, vitamin B_6)
- 2 cups quinoa salad with roasted chickpeas and a lemon-tahini dressing (protein, magnesium, vitamin B_6)
- 6-ounce spinach and feta–stuffed chicken breast with a side of quinoa (protein, vitamin B_6, vitamin B_9)
- 2 grilled vegetable and tofu skewers with brown rice (protein, magnesium, vitamin B_6)
- 3 ounces grilled salmon on a bed of salad made with 2 cups spinach, ½ small avocado, sliced, and a citrus vinaigrette (omega-3s, potassium, vitamin D)
- 6-ounce grilled boneless, skinless chicken breast with ½ cup steamed broccoli and ½ cup quinoa (protein, fiber, magnesium)

- 1½ cups lentil soup with a side of mixed greens (fiber, folate)
- 2 cups quinoa and chickpea salad with spinach and tahini dressing (fiber, magnesium)
- 2 cups spinach and kale salad with grilled tofu and balsamic vinaigrette (fiber, folate)
- 2 cups of black bean and vegetable burrito bowl with 1 cup brown rice (fiber, folate, potassium)
- 6 ounces grilled salmon with ½ cup quinoa and ½ cup steamed broccoli (omega-3s, magnesium, vitamin B_6, vitamin B_9)
- Whole-grain wrap with grilled tofu, avocado, and mixed greens (fiber, protein, vitamin B_6, vitamin B_9)
- 2 cups quinoa salad with chickpeas, cucumbers, and feta cheese (protein, calcium, vitamin B_9)
- 2 cups spinach and mixed bean salad with a lemon-tahini dressing (fiber, magnesium, vitamin B_6, vitamin B_9)
- 2 cups quinoa and black bean bowl with avocado and salsa (fiber, potassium, vitamin B_9)
- 2 cups lentil and vegetable soup (fiber, vitamin B_9)
- 1 large quinoa and black bean–stuffed pepper (fiber, potassium, vitamin B_6, vitamin B_9)

DINNER

- 6-ounce grilled or baked boneless, skinless chicken breast with 1 cup side salad (vitamin B_6, vitamin B_9, calcium, fiber)
- 6 ounces grilled tofu with ½ cup brown rice and ½ cup sautéed kale (protein, magnesium, vitamin B_{12})
- 6 grilled shrimp with 4 medium asparagus spears and ½ cup quinoa (protein, magnesium, vitamin B_6)
- 6 ounces baked cod with 1 small baked sweet potato and ½ cup green beans (protein, vitamin B_6, vitamin B_9)
- 2 cups beef stew with carrots, potatoes, and peas (protein, vitamin B_6, vitamin B_9)
- 6 ounces grilled mackerel with ½ cup quinoa and ½ cup sautéed spinach (protein, omega-3s, magnesium)

- 6 ounces baked trout with ½ cup brown rice and 4 medium steamed asparagus spears (protein, omega-3s, vitamin D)
- 6 ounces roasted chicken with 1 small baked sweet potato and ½ cup steamed broccoli (protein, vitamin B_6, vitamin D)
- 6 ounces baked cod with ½ cup quinoa and 1 cup roasted Brussels sprouts (protein, vitamin B_6, vitamin B_9)
- 2 beef and vegetable kebabs with ½ cup couscous (protein, vitamin B_6, vitamin B_9)
- 6 ounces grilled swordfish with ½ cup brown rice and ½ cup sautéed Swiss chard (protein, omega-3s, vitamin D)
- 2 baked chicken thighs with ½ cup wild rice and ½ cup green beans (protein, vitamin B_6, vitamin B_9)
- 6 ounces baked trout with 1 cup sweet potato fries and ½ cup steamed asparagus (protein, omega-3s, vitamin D)
- 2 cups beef and vegetable stir-fry with a ginger soy sauce (protein, magnesium, vitamin B_6)
- 1 large quinoa-stuffed bell peppers with black beans and tomatoes (fiber, magnesium, folate)
- 6 ounces baked cod with 4 medium asparagus spears and ½ cup brown rice (omega-3s, potassium)
- 2 cups tofu stir-fry with broccoli, bell peppers, and ½ cup brown rice (protein, magnesium)
- 6 grilled shrimp with 1 sweet potato and ½ cup steamed broccoli (protein, potassium)
- 2 baked chicken thighs with quinoa and roasted Brussels sprouts (protein, folate)
- 6 ounces baked salmon with 4 medium asparagus spears and ½ cup quinoa (omega-3s, potassium)
- 6 ounces grilled sirloin steak with 1 cup sweet potato fries and ½ cup steamed broccoli (protein, vitamin B_6)
- 2 cups whole-wheat pasta with spinach, tomatoes, and extra-virgin olive oil (fiber, vitamin B_6)
- 2 cups whole-wheat spaghetti with sautéed kale, garlic, and extra-virgin olive oil (fiber, vitamin B_6)

- 6 ounces grilled salmon with 1 small baked sweet potato and ½ cup steamed broccoli (omega-3s, magnesium, vitamin B_6)
- 4 shrimp and vegetable stir-fry with ½ cup brown rice (protein, vitamin B_6)
- 2 cups whole-wheat pasta with 3 ounces grilled chicken, broccoli, and tomato sauce (protein, fiber, vitamin B_6)
- 6-ounce baked boneless, skinless chicken breast with ½ cup quinoa and 4 medium asparagus spears (protein, vitamin B_6)
- 6 grilled shrimp with whole-wheat pasta and 4 medium roasted asparagus spears (protein, vitamin B_6)
- 6 ounces baked cod with quinoa and ½ cup steamed broccoli (omega-3s, magnesium, vitamin B_6)

SNACKS

- ½ cup Greek yogurt parfait (calcium, protein, vitamin B_6, vitamin B_9, vitamin B_{12})
- Almonds (20) (magnesium, fiber, protein, potassium, omega-3s)
- 4 ounces chia pudding with 1 tablespoon chia seeds (fiber, omega-3s, calcium, magnesium)
- 2 cups spinach and kale salad (fiber, magnesium, calcium, vitamin B_6, vitamin B_9, vitamin B_{12})
- 2 hard-boiled eggs (protein, vitamin B_6, vitamin B_{12}, omega-3s)
- ½ cup cottage cheese with pineapple (protein, calcium, vitamin B_{12})
- 1 cup edamame (protein, fiber, magnesium, vitamin B_6)
- 2 ounces smoked salmon (omega-3s, vitamin D, vitamin B_6, vitamin B_9, vitamin B_{12})
- ¼ cup sunflower seeds (magnesium, fiber, protein, potassium, vitamin B_6)
- 1 cup fortified cereal with ½ cup milk (calcium, vitamin B_6, vitamin B_9, vitamin B_{12}, vitamin D)
- 2 cups kale chips (fiber, calcium, vitamin B_6, magnesium)

- 2 ounces sardines on whole-wheat crackers (omega-3s, vitamin D, vitamin B_{12}, calcium)
- 1 medium kiwi and ½ cup cottage cheese (vitamin C, calcium, protein, vitamin B_6, vitamin B_{12})
- 1 cup quinoa salad with black beans and avocado (fiber, magnesium, protein, vitamin B_6, potassium)
- 1 cup mixed berries and 1 tablespoon almond butter (fiber, omega-3s, magnesium, vitamin B_6, vitamin B_9)
- ½ cup roasted chickpeas (protein, fiber, magnesium, vitamin B_6, potassium)
- 4 medium walnut and spinach–stuffed mushrooms) (omega-3s, magnesium, calcium, vitamin B_6, vitamin B_9)
- 1 cup tuna salad in lettuce wraps (protein, vitamin B_6, vitamin B_{12}, omega-3s, magnesium)
- 1 medium orange and 1 ounce dark chocolate (vitamin C, fiber, magnesium, potassium, iron, antioxidants)
- ¼ cup pumpkin seeds (magnesium, protein, fiber, potassium)

30-DAY MEAL PLAN

DAY 1

Breakfast
- 8 ounces Greek yogurt with berries and 1 teaspoon honey, sprinkled with 1 tablespoon chia seeds (calcium, fiber, protein, omega-3s)

Lunch
- 6 ounces grilled salmon with ½ cup quinoa and ½ cup steamed broccoli (protein, omega-3s, magnesium, fiber)

Snack
- 20 almonds, 1 medium orange (potassium, magnesium)

Dinner
- 6-ounce grilled or baked boneless, skinless chicken breast with 1 cup side salad (vitamin B_6, vitamin B_9, calcium, fiber)

DAY 2

Breakfast
- 1½ cups oatmeal topped with ¼ small banana, sliced, and ¼ cup walnuts (fiber, magnesium, potassium)

Lunch
- 1½ cups lentil soup and 1 cup spinach salad (protein, fiber, magnesium, vitamin B_6, vitamin B_9)

Snack
- 1 small carrot, sliced, or 1 small cucumber, sliced, with 2 tablespoons hummus (fiber)

Dinner
- Grilled tofu with ½ cup brown rice and ½ cup sautéed kale (protein, magnesium, vitamin B_{12})

DAY 3

Breakfast
- 1 slice whole-grain toast with ½ small avocado, mashed, and 2 poached eggs (fiber, vitamin D, vitamin B_{12})

Lunch
- 2 cups quinoa and black bean salad with a side of ¼ cup guacamole (protein, magnesium, vitamin B_{12})

Snack
- ¼ cup low-fat cottage cheese and ¼ cup pineapple slices (calcium, vitamin B_{12})

Dinner
- 6 grilled shrimp with 4 medium asparagus spears and ½ cup quinoa (protein, magnesium, vitamin B_6)

DAY 4

Breakfast
- 2-egg spinach and feta omelet (protein, calcium, vitamin B_6, vitamin B_{12})

Lunch
- ½ cup tuna salad with ½ cup mixed greens and 8 whole-grain crackers (omega-3s, vitamin D)

Snack
- ½ cup mixed nuts and 1 medium pear (fiber, protein, potassium, magnesium, monounsaturated fats)

Dinner
- 6 ounces baked cod with 1 small baked sweet potato and ½ cup green beans (protein, vitamin B_6, vitamin B_9)

DAY 5

Breakfast
- 12-ounce smoothie made with milk or juice, spinach, banana, and flaxseeds (fiber, potassium, vitamin B_6)

Lunch
- 2 cups chickpea and vegetable stir-fry with ½ cup brown rice (protein, magnesium, vitamin B_6)

Snack
- ½ cup cottage cheese with sliced strawberries (calcium, vitamin B_{12})

Dinner
- 2 cups beef stew with carrots, potatoes, and peas (protein, vitamin B_6, vitamin B_9)

DAY 6

Breakfast
- 2 small whole-grain pancakes with fresh blueberries (fiber, vitamin B_6, vitamin B_9)

Lunch
- Turkey and avocado wrap with a side of mixed greens (protein, vitamin B_6, magnesium)

Snack
- 1 cup sliced bell peppers with 2 tablespoons hummus (fiber)

Dinner
- 6 ounces grilled mackerel with ½ cup quinoa and ½ cup sautéed spinach (protein, omega-3s, magnesium)

DAY 7

Breakfast
- 1 cup low-fat cottage cheese and mixed fruit salad (calcium, vitamin B_{12})

Lunch
- 2 cups spinach and kale salad with 6-ounce grilled boneless, skinless chicken breast (protein, vitamin B_6, vitamin B_9)

Snack
- ¼ cup almond and cranberry trail mix (potassium, magnesium)

Dinner
- 6 ounces baked trout with ½ cup brown rice and 4 medium steamed asparagus spears (protein, omega-3s, vitamin D)

DAY 8

Breakfast
- 2 scrambled eggs with sautéed spinach and 1 slice whole-grain toast (protein, vitamin B_6, vitamin B_9)

Lunch
- 6 ounces grilled tilapia with 1 cup quinoa and a mixed greens salad (protein, omega-3s, magnesium)

Snack
- ½ cup Greek yogurt with honey and sliced almonds (calcium, vitamin B_{12})

Dinner
- 6 ounces roasted chicken with 1 small baked sweet potato and ½ cup steamed broccoli (protein, vitamin B$_6$, vitamin D)

DAY 9

Breakfast
- 2 small or 1 large whole-grain waffle with strawberries and a drizzle of maple syrup (fiber, vitamin B$_6$, vitamin B$_9$)

Lunch
- 2 cups black bean and corn salad with 3 grilled shrimp (protein, magnesium, vitamin B$_6$)

Snack
- 1 small cucumber, sliced, and 5 cherry tomatoes with 2 tablespoons tzatziki (fiber)

Dinner
- 6 ounces baked cod with ½ cup quinoa and 1 cup roasted Brussels sprouts (protein, vitamin B$_6$, vitamin B$_9$)

DAY 10

Breakfast
- 1½ cups overnight oats with 1 tablespoon almond butter, ¼ small banana, and 1 teaspoon chia seeds (fiber, magnesium, potassium)

Lunch
- 2 cups turkey and vegetable stir-fry with ½ cup brown rice (protein, magnesium, vitamin B$_6$)

Snack
- ¼ cup mixed nuts and 1 medium apple (fiber, potassium, magnesium, monounsaturated fats)

Dinner
- 2 beef and vegetable kebabs with a side of ½ cup couscous (protein, vitamin B$_6$, vitamin B$_9$)

DAY 11

Breakfast
- 12-ounce smoothie made with milk or juice, kale, pineapple, Greek yogurt, and flaxseeds (fiber, calcium, vitamin B_6)

Lunch
- 1½ cups lentil and vegetable curry with 1 piece of whole-grain naan (protein, magnesium, vitamin B_6)

Snack
- 1 cup celery or carrot sticks with peanut butter (fiber)

Dinner
- 6 ounces grilled swordfish with ½ cup brown rice and ½ cup sautéed Swiss chard (protein, omega-3s, vitamin D)

DAY 12

Breakfast
- ½ small avocado, sliced, and 3 ounces smoked salmon on 1 slice whole-grain toast (omega-3s, vitamin D, vitamin B_{12})

Lunch
- 2 cups quinoa salad with roasted chickpeas and a lemon tahini dressing (protein, magnesium, vitamin B_6)

Snack
- 6 ounces low-fat yogurt with mixed berries (calcium, vitamin B_{12})

Dinner
- 2 baked chicken thighs with ½ cup wild rice and ½ cup green beans (protein, vitamin B_6, vitamin B_9)

DAY 13

Breakfast
- 1 cup low-fat cottage cheese with sliced peaches and a sprinkle of almonds (calcium, vitamin B_{12})

Lunch
- 6-ounce spinach and feta–stuffed chicken breast with ½ cup quinoa (protein, vitamin B_6, vitamin B_9)

Snack
- Trail mix with dried apricots (potassium, magnesium)

Dinner
- 6 ounces baked trout with 1 small baked sweet potato fries and 4 medium steamed asparagus spears (protein, omega-3s, vitamin D)

DAY 14

Breakfast
- 1 cup whole-grain cereal with almond milk and sliced strawberries (fiber, vitamin B_6, vitamin B_9)

Lunch
- 2 grilled vegetable and tofu skewers with 1 cup brown rice (protein, magnesium, vitamin B_6)

Snack
- 1 small bell pepper, sliced, with 2 tablespoons hummus (fiber)

Dinner
- 2 cups beef and vegetable stir-fry with a ginger soy sauce (protein, magnesium, vitamin B_6)

DAY 15

Breakfast
- 8 ounces Greek yogurt with mixed berries and 1 tablespoon chia seeds (calcium, fiber, protein, omega-3s, vitamin B_6)

Snack
- 20 almonds (magnesium, protein)

Lunch
- 6 ounces grilled salmon salad with spinach, avocado, and a citrus vinaigrette (omega-3s, potassium, vitamin D)

Snack
- 1 cup carrot sticks with 2 tablespoons hummus (fiber, vitamin B_6)

Dinner
- 1 large quinoa-stuffed bell pepper with black beans and tomatoes (fiber, magnesium, folate)

Dessert
- 1 cup low-fat milk or fortified almond milk (calcium, vitamin B_{12})

DAY 16

Breakfast
- 1½ cups oatmeal with ¼ small banana, sliced, and ¼ cup walnuts (fiber, potassium, magnesium)

Snack
- ½ cup Greek yogurt with honey and flaxseeds (calcium, protein, omega-3s)

Lunch
- 6-ounce grilled boneless, skinless chicken breast with ½ cup steamed broccoli and ½ cup quinoa (protein, fiber, magnesium)

Snack
- 1 cup edamame (protein, magnesium)

Dinner
- 6 ounces baked cod with 4 medium asparagus spears and ½ cup brown rice (omega-3s, potassium)

Dessert
- 6 ounces fortified yogurt with sliced strawberries (calcium, vitamin B_6)

DAY 17

Breakfast
- 2-egg spinach and feta omelet with 1 slice whole-grain toast (protein, folate)

Snack
- ½ cup mixed nuts (fiber, magnesium, monounsaturated fats, protein)

Lunch
- 1½ cups lentil soup with a side of mixed greens (fiber, folate)

Snack
- 1 medium orange (vitamin C, potassium)

Dinner
- 2 cups tofu stir-fry with broccoli, bell peppers, and ½ cup brown rice (protein, magnesium)

Dessert
- 1 cup fortified orange juice (vitamin D, vitamin B_{12})

DAY 18

Breakfast
- 1½ cups whole-grain cereal with milk and sliced strawberries (calcium, fiber, vitamin D)

Snack
- ½ cup cottage cheese with ¼ cup pineapple chunks (calcium, protein)

Lunch
- 2 cups quinoa and chickpea salad with spinach and tahini dressing (fiber, magnesium)

Snack
- 1 cup celery sticks with 1 tablespoon peanut butter (protein, magnesium)

Dinner
- 6 grilled shrimp with 1 baked sweet potato and ½ cup steamed broccoli (protein, potassium)

Dessert
- 1 cup almond milk with 1 banana (vitamin B_6, vitamin B_{12})

DAY 19

Breakfast
- 12-ounce smoothie made with milk or juice, kale, banana, chia seeds, and almond milk (fiber, potassium, omega-3s)

Snack
- ¼ cup pumpkin seeds (magnesium, protein)

Lunch
- Turkey and avocado wrap with whole-grain tortilla (protein, vitamin B_6)

Snack
- 1 cup mixed berries (fiber, vitamin C)

Dinner
- 2 baked chicken thighs with ½ cup quinoa and 1 cup roasted Brussels sprouts (protein, folate)

Dessert
- 6 ounces yogurt with kiwi (calcium, vitamin B_{12})

DAY 20

Breakfast
- 2 cottage cheese pancakes with blueberries (calcium, protein, fiber)

Snack
- ⅓ cup trail mix with dried fruits and nuts (magnesium, protein)

Lunch
- 2 cups spinach and kale salad with grilled tofu and balsamic vinaigrette (fiber, folate)

Snack
- 1 small cucumber, sliced, with tzatziki (calcium, vitamin B_6)

Dinner
- 6 ounces baked salmon with 4 medium asparagus spears and quinoa (omega-3s, potassium)

Dessert
- 1 cup fortified orange juice (vitamin D, vitamin B_{12})

DAY 21

Breakfast
- 2 small or 1 large whole-grain waffle with strawberries and a drizzle of honey (fiber, potassium)

Snack
- 6 ounces low-fat yogurt with almonds and raspberries (calcium, protein, magnesium)

Lunch
- 2 cups black bean and vegetable burrito bowl with 1 cup brown rice (fiber, folate, potassium)

Snack
- 1 cup carrots with 2 tablespoons guacamole (fiber, vitamin B_6)

Dinner
- 6-ounce grilled sirloin steak with 1 cup sweet potato fries and ½ cup steamed broccoli (protein, vitamin B_6)

Dessert
- 1 cup fortified almond milk with a handful of walnuts (calcium, omega-3s)

DAY 22

Breakfast
- 8 ounces Greek yogurt with berries and almonds (calcium, protein, fiber)

Lunch
- 6 ounces grilled salmon with ½ cup quinoa and ½ cup steamed broccoli (omega-3s, magnesium, vitamin B_6, vitamin B_9)

Snack
- 1 cup carrot sticks with 2 tablespoons hummus (fiber, magnesium)

Dinner
- 2 cups whole-wheat pasta with spinach, tomatoes, and extra-virgin olive oil (fiber, vitamin B_6)

Snack
- ½ cup low-fat cottage cheese with pineapple (calcium, vitamin B_{12})

DAY 23

Breakfast
- 2-egg spinach and feta omelet (protein, calcium, vitamin B_6, vitamin B_{12})

Lunch
- Whole-grain wrap with grilled tofu, avocado, and mixed greens (fiber, protein, vitamin B_6, vitamin B_9)

Snack
- 1 small bell pepper with 2 tablespoons guacamole (fiber, potassium)

Dinner
- 2 cups whole-wheat spaghetti with sautéed kale, garlic, and extra-virgin olive oil (fiber, vitamin B_6)

Snack
- 1 cup berries and a handful of walnuts (omega-3s, vitamin B_9)

DAY 24

Breakfast
- 12-ounce smoothie made with milk or juice, kale, banana, and flaxseeds (fiber, potassium, vitamin B_6, vitamin B_9)

Lunch
- 2 cups quinoa salad with chickpeas, cucumbers, and feta cheese (protein, calcium, vitamin B_9)

Snack
- ½ cup Greek yogurt with honey (calcium, vitamin B_{12})

Dinner
- 6 ounces grilled salmon with 1 small baked sweet potato and ½ cup steamed broccoli (omega-3s, magnesium, vitamin B_6)

Snack
- ½ cup low-fat cottage cheese and sliced strawberries (calcium, vitamin B_9)

DAY 25

Breakfast
- 1½ cups whole-grain cereal with low-fat milk (calcium, vitamin B_{12})

Lunch
- 2 cups spinach and mixed bean salad with a lemon-tahini dressing (fiber, magnesium, vitamin B_6, vitamin B_9)

Snack
- ¼ cup almonds and 3 dried apricots (magnesium, potassium)

Dinner
- 4 shrimp and 1 cup vegetable stir-fry with ½ cup brown rice (protein, vitamin B_6)

Snack
- 1 medium pear, sliced, with a handful of walnuts (fiber, omega-3s, vitamin B_9)

DAY 26

Breakfast
- 2 scrambled eggs with sautéed spinach and 1 slice whole-grain toast (protein, fiber, vitamin B_6, vitamin B_9)

Lunch
- 2 cups quinoa and black bean bowl with avocado and salsa (fiber, potassium, vitamin B_9)

Snack
- 1 cup carrots with 2 tablespoons tzatziki sauce (calcium, fiber)

Dinner
- 2 cups whole-wheat pasta with 6 ounces grilled chicken, ½ cup broccoli, and tomato sauce (protein, fiber, vitamin B_6)

Snack
- 6 ounces low-fat yogurt with mixed berries (calcium, vitamin B_{12})

DAY 27

Breakfast
- 1½ cups oatmeal with 1 tablespoon chia seeds, ¼ small banana, and 1 tablespoon almond butter (fiber, magnesium, potassium, vitamin B_6)

Lunch
- 1½ cups lentil and vegetable soup (fiber, vitamin B_9)

Snack
- ½ cup mixed nuts (fiber, protein, monounsaturated fats, magnesium, omega-3s)

Dinner
- 6-ounce baked boneless, skinless chicken breast with ½ cup quinoa and 4 medium asparagus spears (protein, vitamin B_6)

Snack
- 6 ounces low-fat yogurt (calcium, vitamin B_{12})

DAY 28

Breakfast
- 1 cup cottage cheese with sliced peaches and a sprinkle of flaxseeds (calcium, fiber, vitamin B_{12})

Lunch
- 1 large quinoa and black bean–stuffed peppers (fiber, potassium, vitamin B_6, vitamin B_9)

Snack
- ¼ cup mixed nuts and dried apricots (fiber, protein, monounsaturated fats, magnesium, omega-3s)

Dinner

- 4 grilled shrimp with 2 cups whole-wheat pasta and roasted aspar-agus (protein, vitamin B$_6$)

Snack

- ½ cup Greek yogurt with honey and blueberries (calcium, vita-min B$_{12}$)

DAY 29

Breakfast

- 2 small or 1 whole-grain waffle with 1 tablespoon almond butter and sliced strawberries (fiber, magnesium, vitamin B$_6$, vitamin B$_9$)

Lunch

- 1 cup lentil soup with 1 cup mixed greens and a lemon-tahini dress-ing (fiber, magnesium, vitamin B$_6$, vitamin B$_9$)

Snack

- 1 small cucumber, sliced, with 2 tablespoons tzatziki sauce (calcium, fiber)

Dinner

- 2 baked chicken thighs with ½ cup sweet potato mash and ½ cup steamed green beans (protein, vitamin B$_6$)

Snack

- 1 cup mixed berries and a handful of walnuts (omega-3s, vitamin B$_9$)

DAY 30

Breakfast

- 1½ cups overnight oats with almond milk, chia seeds, and mixed berries (fiber, magnesium, vitamin B$_6$, vitamin B$_9$)

Lunch

- Turkey and avocado whole-grain wrap (protein, fiber, vitamin B$_6$, vitamin B$_9$)

Snack
- ¼ cup mixed nuts and dried cranberries (fiber, protein, magnesium, monounsaturated fats, omega-3s)

Dinner
- 6 ounces baked cod with ½ cup quinoa and ½ cup steamed broccoli (omega-3s, magnesium, vitamin B_6)

Snack
- 6 ounces low-fat yogurt with sliced peaches (calcium, vitamin B_{12})

5

RECIPES FOR HEALTHY LIVING

In this chapter you will find some simple, healthy, tasty recipes for breakfast, lunch, and dinner. The number of ingredients in these recipes is purposefully small to make the meals affordable, convenient, and easy to prepare. However, feel free to swap ingredients or expand the recipes to suit your taste, food availability, or nutrient profile preference. While there are lots of power nutrients in each recipe, I have only listed the nutritional info for the macros—carbohydrates, fats, and proteins (as these three are what our bodies need in large supply)—and fiber. These recipes are just a blueprint, and what you ultimately decide to create from them is all up to you. These meals have been designed so that you can enjoy them at any decade of your life and benefit from all of their health-promoting ingredients. Enjoy!

AVOCADO TOAST WITH POACHED EGGS

SERVES 2

2 slices whole-grain bread

1 ripe avocado, pit removed

2 eggs

Salt and pepper to taste

Toast the bread slices until golden brown.

Mash the avocado and spread it evenly on the toast.

Poach the eggs until the whites are set but the yolks are still runny. Place 1 poached egg on top of each slice of the avocado toast. Season with salt and pepper.

Nutritional Info (per serving): *Calories: 320; Protein: 13g; Carbohydrates: 26g; Fat: 20g; Fiber: 8g*

GREEK YOGURT PARFAIT

SERVES 1

1 cup Greek yogurt

½ cup granola

½ cup mixed berries (strawberries, blueberries, raspberries)

Honey (optional)

In a glass or bowl, layer the Greek yogurt, granola, and mixed berries.

Repeat the layers until ingredients are used up.

Drizzle honey on top if desired.

Nutritional Info (per serving): *Calories: 350; Protein: 18g; Carbohydrates: 45g; Fat: 10g; Fiber: 6g*

SPINACH AND MUSHROOM OMELET

SERVES 1

1 teaspoon extra-virgin olive oil

½ cup spinach leaves

¼ cup sliced mushrooms

2 eggs

Salt and pepper to taste

Heat a nonstick skillet over medium heat. Add the olive oil and heat until the oil is shimmering.

Add the spinach and mushrooms to the skillet and sauté until tender, about 5 minutes.

In a small bowl, beat the eggs. Season with salt and pepper.

Pour the beaten eggs into the skillet over the spinach and mushrooms.

Cook until the eggs are set, then fold the omelet in half and serve.

Nutritional Info (per serving): *Calories: 220; Protein: 16g; Carbohydrates: 4g; Fat: 16g; Fiber 3g*

QUINOA BREAKFAST BOWL

SERVES 1

½ cup quinoa

¼ cup almonds, sliced

½ cup diced apple

1 tablespoon honey

Cinnamon to taste

Cook the quinoa according to package instructions.

In a bowl, combine the cooked quinoa, sliced almonds, diced apple, honey, and cinnamon.

Stir well to combine.

Nutritional info (per serving): *Calories: 320; Protein: 9g; Carbohydrates: 50g; Fat: 10g; Fiber: 8g*

VEGGIE BREAKFAST BURRITO

SERVES 2

1 teaspoon extra-virgin olive oil

2 eggs

2 whole-wheat tortillas

½ cup black beans, rinsed and drained

¼ cup diced bell peppers

¼ cup diced onion

¼ cup shredded cheddar cheese

Salsa or hot sauce (optional)

Heat a nonstick skillet on medium heat. Add the olive oil.

In a small bowl, beat the eggs.

Pour the beaten eggs into the skillet and cook until soft.

Remove the scrambled eggs and set aside.

Wipe the skillet clean and return to medium heat.

Add 1 tortilla and heat for 2 minutes on each side. Repeat with the second tortilla.

Fill each tortilla with half of the scrambled eggs, black beans, bell peppers, onion, and cheese.

Roll up the tortillas to form burritos.

Serve with salsa or hot sauce if desired.

Nutritional info (per serving): *Calories: 380; Protein: 21g; Carbohydrates: 40g; Fat: 16g; Fiber: 10g*

OVERNIGHT OATS WITH CHIA SEEDS AND BERRIES

SERVES 1

½ cup rolled oats

1 tablespoon chia seeds

½ cup almond milk

1 tablespoon honey or maple syrup (optional)

¼ teaspoon vanilla extract

½ cup mixed berries (strawberries, blueberries, raspberries)

In a mason jar or airtight container, combine the rolled oats, chia seeds, almond milk, honey or maple syrup (if using), and vanilla extract.

Stir well to combine all the ingredients.

Add the mixed berries on top of the oat mixture.

Seal the jar or container and refrigerate overnight or at least 4 hours.

In the morning, give the oats a good stir before eating.

Enjoy cold, or warm up by heating in the microwave, lid off, for 1 to 2 minutes if desired.

Nutritional Info (per serving): *Calories: 320; Protein: 10g; Carbohydrates: 54g; Fat: 8g; Fiber: 12g*

SWEET POTATO AND SPINACH BREAKFAST HASH

SERVES 2

1 tablespoon extra-virgin olive oil

1 large sweet potato, peeled and diced

¼ cup diced onion

1 garlic clove, minced

2 cups fresh spinach leaves

2 eggs

Salt and pepper to taste

Heat the olive oil in a skillet over medium heat.

Add the diced sweet potato to the skillet and cook, stirring frequently, until softened and lightly browned, 8 to 10 minutes.

Add the diced onion to the skillet and cook, about 5 minutes until translucent.

Add the minced garlic to the skillet and cook about 1 minute until fragrant.

Stir in the fresh spinach leaves and cook until wilted, 2 to 3 minutes.

Create two wells in the hash mixture and crack an egg into each well.

Cover the skillet and cook until the eggs are cooked to your desired level of doneness, 3 to 4 minutes for runny yolks.

Season with salt and pepper before serving.

Nutritional Info (per serving): *Calories: 280; Protein: 10g; Carbohydrates: 30g; Fat: 14g; Fiber: 5g*

BERRY PROTEIN SMOOTHIE BOWL

SERVES 1

1 cup mixed berries
(strawberries, blueberries,
raspberries)

½ banana

½ cup Greek yogurt

1 scoop protein powder (vanilla
or berry flavor)

¼ cup almond milk

Toppings: sliced almonds,
shredded coconut, chia
seeds

In a blender, combine the mixed berries, banana, Greek yogurt, protein powder, and almond milk.

Blend until smooth and creamy.

Pour the smoothie into a bowl.

Top with sliced almonds, shredded coconut, and chia seeds.

Serve immediately.

Nutritional Info (per serving): *Calories: 380; Protein: 30g; Carbohydrates: 45g; Fat: 12g; Fiber: 10g*

VEGGIE BREAKFAST CASSEROLE

SERVES 4

Cooking spray or extra-virgin olive oil for greasing the baking dish

6 eggs

½ cup diced bell peppers

½ cup diced onion

1 cup diced tomatoes

1 cup chopped spinach

½ cup shredded cheddar cheese

Salt and pepper to taste

Preheat the oven to 350°F (175°C). Lightly grease a baking dish with cooking spray or olive oil.

In a large bowl, beat the eggs until well combined.

Stir in the bell peppers, onion, tomatoes, spinach, and cheese.

Season with salt and pepper.

Pour the egg mixture into the prepared baking dish.

Bake in the preheated oven for 25 to 30 minutes, or until the eggs are set and the top is golden brown.

Allow the casserole to cool for a few minutes before slicing and serving.

Nutritional Info (per serving): *Calories: 180; Protein: 14g; Carbohydrates: 6g; Fat: 11g; Fiber: 2g*

BANANA ALMOND BUTTER PROTEIN PANCAKES

SERVES 2

1 ripe banana, mashed

2 eggs

2 tablespoons almond butter

¼ teaspoon ground cinnamon

¼ teaspoon baking powder

Cooking spray or coconut oil for greasing the skillet

In a bowl, mash the ripe banana until smooth.

Add the eggs, almond butter, cinnamon, and baking powder to the bowl and whisk until well combined.

Heat a skillet over medium heat and lightly grease it with cooking spray or coconut oil.

Pour about ¼ cup of the pancake batter into the skillet for each pancake.

Cook for 2 to 3 minutes on each side, or until golden brown.

Repeat with the remaining batter.

Serve the pancakes warm with your favorite toppings such as sliced bananas, berries, or a drizzle of honey.

Nutritional Info (per serving): *Calories: 320; Protein: 15g; Carbohydrates: 20g; Fat: 20g; Fiber: 4g*

TOFU SCRAMBLE WITH VEGETABLES

SERVES 2

Cooking spray or extra-virgin olive oil for greasing the skillet

¼ cup diced bell peppers

¼ cup diced onion

½ block firm tofu, drained and crumbled

¼ cup diced tomatoes

½ cup chopped spinach

1 tablespoon nutritional yeast (optional)

½ teaspoon turmeric powder

Salt and pepper to taste

Heat a skillet over medium heat and lightly grease it with cooking spray or olive oil.

Add the bell peppers and onion to the skillet and sauté until softened, 3 to 4 minutes.

Add the tofu, tomatoes, spinach, nutritional yeast (if using), turmeric powder, salt, and pepper to the skillet.

Cook for another 5 to 6 minutes, stirring occasionally, until the tofu is heated through and the vegetables are tender.

Adjust seasoning to taste before serving.

Nutritional Info (per serving): *Calories: 150; Protein: 14g; Carbohydrates: 10g; Fat: 7g; Fiber: 3g*

QUINOA SALAD WITH CHICKPEAS AND AVOCADO

SERVES 4

1 cup quinoa, cooked

1 (15-ounce) can chickpeas, drained and rinsed

1 avocado, diced

1 cup cherry tomatoes, halved

¼ cup chopped fresh cilantro

2 tablespoons extra-virgin olive oil

2 tablespoons freshly squeezed lemon juice

Salt and pepper to taste

Cook the quinoa according to package instructions and let it cool.

In a large bowl, combine the cooked quinoa, chickpeas, avocado, cherry tomatoes, and cilantro.

In a small bowl, whisk together the olive oil and lemon juice. Season with salt and pepper.

Pour the dressing over the salad and toss gently to combine.

Serve immediately or refrigerate until ready to eat.

Nutritional Info (per serving): *Calories: 350; Protein: 10g; Carbohydrates: 45g; Fat: 15 g; Fiber: 9g*

GRILLED CHICKEN AND VEGETABLE WRAP

SERVES 4

2 boneless, skinless chicken breasts

1 red bell pepper, sliced

1 yellow bell pepper, sliced

1 zucchini, sliced

1 tablespoon extra-virgin olive oil

Salt and pepper to taste

4 whole-wheat tortillas

¼ cup hummus

Preheat the grill to medium-high heat.

Brush the chicken breasts and vegetables with the olive oil and season with salt and pepper.

Grill the chicken breasts for 6 to 8 minutes per side, or until cooked through, and grill the vegetables until tender.

Slice the chicken into strips.

Warm the tortillas, then spread hummus evenly over each one and top with a quarter of the chicken and vegetables.

Roll up the tortillas tightly and cut the wraps in half before serving.

Nutritional Info (per serving): *Calories: 320; Protein: 25g; Carbohydrates: 30g; Fat: 12 g; Fiber: 7g*

LENTIL SOUP

SERVES 6

2 tablespoons extra-virgin olive oil

1 onion, chopped

2 carrots, diced

2 stalks celery, diced

3 cloves garlic, minced

1 cup dried green lentils, sorted and rinsed

6 cups vegetable broth

1 teaspoon dried thyme

1 teaspoon dried oregano

Salt and pepper to taste

In a large stockpot, heat the olive oil over medium heat.

Add the onion, carrots, and celery. Cook until the vegetables are softened, about 5 minutes.

Add the garlic and cook for about 1 minute until fragrant.

Add the lentils, vegetable broth, thyme, and oregano. Season with salt and pepper.

Bring to a boil, then reduce heat and simmer for 25 to 30 minutes, or until lentils are tender.

Adjust seasoning if necessary.

Serve hot.

Nutritional Info (per serving): *Calories: 220; Protein: 12g; Carbohydrates: 32g; Fat: 5g; Fiber: 15g*

GREEK SALAD WITH GRILLED SHRIMP

SERVES 4

1 pound large shrimp, peeled and deveined

6 cups mixed salad greens

1 cucumber, diced

1 cup cherry tomatoes, halved

½ red onion, thinly sliced

½ cup pitted Kalamata olives

¼ cup crumbled feta cheese

2 tablespoons extra-virgin olive oil

2 tablespoons red wine vinegar

1 teaspoon dried oregano

Salt and pepper to taste

Preheat grill to medium-high heat.

Thread shrimp onto skewers and grill for 2 to 3 minutes per side, or until pink and cooked through. Set aside.

In a large bowl, combine the salad greens, cucumber, cherry tomatoes, red onion, olives, and feta cheese.

In a small bowl, whisk together the olive oil, red wine vinegar, and oregano. Season with salt and pepper.

Pour the dressing over the salad and toss to coat.

Divide the salad onto plates and top with the grilled shrimp.

Nutritional Info (per serving): *Calories: 280; Protein: 25g; Carbohydrates: 10g; Fat: 15 g; Fiber: 3g*

VEGGIE STIR-FRY WITH TOFU

SERVES 4

2 tablespoons soy sauce

3 tablespoons sesame oil,
plus more as needed

1 tablespoon cornstarch

¼ cup water

1 (14-ounce) block firm tofu,
pressed and cubed

2 cups broccoli florets

1 red bell pepper, sliced

1 yellow bell pepper, sliced

1 carrot, julienned

1 cup snap peas

2 cloves garlic, minced

Cooked brown rice for serving

In a small bowl, whisk together the soy sauce, 1 tablespoon sesame oil, cornstarch, and water. Set aside.

Add the remaining 2 tablespoons of sesame oil to a large skillet or wok and warm over medium-high heat. Add the tofu cubes and cook until golden brown on all sides. Remove the tofu from the skillet and set aside.

In the same skillet, add a little more oil if needed. Add the broccoli, bell peppers, carrot, snap peas, and garlic. Stir-fry for 3 to 4 minutes, or until vegetables are tender-crisp.

Return the tofu to the skillet and pour the sauce over the tofu and vegetables. Cook for another 2 to 3 minutes, or until the sauce has thickened.

Serve hot over cooked brown rice.

Nutritional Info (per serving): *Calories: 280; Protein: 18g; Carbohydrates: 25g; Fat: 13 g; Fiber: 6g*

TURKEY AND HUMMUS WRAP

SERVES 4

4 whole-wheat wraps

¼ cup hummus

8 slices deli turkey

1 cup mixed salad greens

½ cucumber, thinly sliced

¼ cup shredded carrots

Salt and pepper to taste

Lay out the wraps and spread hummus evenly over each one.

Divide the turkey slices among the wraps.

Top each wrap with a quarter of the mixed greens, cucumber slices, and shredded carrots.

Season with salt and pepper to taste.

Roll up the tortillas tightly and cut the wraps in half before serving.

Nutritional Info (per serving): *Calories: 280; Protein: 20g; Carbohydrates: 30g; Fat: 10g; Fiber: 6g*

MEDITERRANEAN CHICKPEA SALAD

SERVES 4

2 (15-ounce) cans chickpeas, drained and rinsed

1 cucumber, diced

1 cup cherry tomatoes, halved

½ red onion, thinly sliced

¼ cup chopped fresh parsley

¼ cup crumbled feta cheese

2 tablespoons extra-virgin olive oil

2 tablespoons freshly squeezed lemon juice

1 teaspoon dried oregano

Salt and pepper to taste

In a large bowl, combine the chickpeas, cucumber, cherry tomatoes, red onion, parsley, and feta cheese.

In a small bowl, whisk together the olive oil, lemon juice, oregano, salt, and pepper.

Pour the dressing over the salad and toss gently to combine.

Serve immediately or refrigerate until ready to eat.

Nutritional Info (per serving): *Calories: 320; Protein: 14g; Carbohydrates: 35g; Fat: 15g; Fiber: 10g*

VEGGIE AND HUMMUS WRAP

SERVES 4

4 whole-wheat wraps

1 cup hummus

2 cups mixed salad greens

1 bell pepper, thinly sliced

½ cup shredded carrots

½ cup alfalfa sprouts

Salt and pepper to taste

Lay out the wraps and spread hummus evenly over each one.

Layer a quarter of the mixed greens, bell pepper, carrots, and alfalfa sprouts on top of the hummus.

Season with salt and pepper to taste.

Roll up the tortillas tightly and slice the wraps in half before serving.

Nutritional Info (per serving): *Calories: 260; Protein: 10g; Carbohydrates: 30g; Fat: 12g; Fiber: 8g*

SALMON QUINOA BOWL

SERVES 2

2 (6-ounce) salmon fillets

Salt and pepper to taste

2 cups cooked quinoa

2 cups mixed baby spinach

1 cucumber, diced

1 avocado, sliced

¼ cup chopped almonds

2 tablespoons extra-virgin olive oil

2 tablespoons balsamic vinegar

Season the salmon fillets with salt and pepper. Bake or grill until cooked through, 10 to 12 minutes. Set aside.

In a large bowl, combine the quinoa, spinach, cucumber, avocado, and almonds.

In a small bowl, whisk together the olive oil and balsamic vinegar.

Pour the dressing over the quinoa salad and toss to combine.

Divide the quinoa salad into two bowls and top each with a cooked salmon fillet.

Nutritional Info (per serving): *Calories: 520; Protein: 35g; Carbohydrates: 35g; Fat: 28g; Fiber: 10g*

BLACK BEAN AND CORN SALAD

SERVES 4

2 cups cooked black beans

1 cup corn kernels (fresh, canned, or frozen)

1 bell pepper, diced

½ red onion, diced

1 jalapeño, seeded and minced

¼ cup chopped fresh cilantro

2 tablespoons freshly squeezed lime juice

1 tablespoon extra-virgin olive oil

Salt and pepper to taste

In a large bowl, combine the black beans, corn kernels, bell pepper, red onion, jalapeño, and cilantro.

In a small bowl, whisk together the lime juice and olive oil. Season with salt and pepper.

Pour the dressing over the salad and toss gently to combine.

Serve immediately or refrigerate until ready to eat.

Nutritional Info (per serving): *Calories: 240; Protein: 9g; Carbohydrates: 40g; Fat: 6g; Fiber: 10g*

ASIAN-FLARED QUINOA STIR-FRY

SERVES 4

1 cup uncooked quinoa

2 cups water or vegetable broth

1 tablespoon sesame oil

2 cloves garlic, minced

1 tablespoon grated fresh ginger

1 red bell pepper, thinly sliced

1 yellow bell pepper, thinly sliced

1 cup snap peas, trimmed

1 carrot, julienned

1 cup mushrooms, sliced

¼ cup low-sodium soy sauce

2 tablespoons rice vinegar

1 tablespoon honey or maple syrup

2 green onions, chopped, for garnish

Sesame seeds, for garnish

In a saucepan, combine the quinoa and the water or vegetable broth. Bring to a boil, then reduce heat to low, cover, and simmer for 15 to 20 minutes, or until quinoa is cooked and water is absorbed. Remove from heat and let it sit covered for 5 minutes. Fluff with a fork.

In a large skillet or wok, heat the sesame oil over medium heat. Add the garlic and ginger. Cook for 1 minute, until fragrant, then set aside.

Add the red and yellow bell peppers, snap peas, carrot, and mushrooms to the skillet. Stir-fry for 5 to 6 minutes, or until the vegetables are tender-crisp.

In a small bowl, whisk together the soy sauce, rice vinegar, and honey or maple syrup.

Add the cooked quinoa to the skillet with the vegetables. Pour the sauce over the quinoa and vegetables. Stir well to combine and coat everything with the sauce. Add the garlic and ginger. Cook for another 2 to 3 minutes until heated through.

Garnish with the green onions and sesame seeds before serving.

Nutritional Info (per serving): *Calories: 290; Protein: 9g; Carbohydrates: 46g; Fat: 8g; Fiber: 7g*

GRILLED SALMON WITH QUINOA AND ROASTED VEGETABLES

SERVES 4

1 cup uncooked quinoa

2 cups sliced mixed vegetables (such as bell peppers, zucchini, and cherry tomatoes)

2 tablespoons extra-virgin olive oil

Salt and pepper to taste

4 salmon fillets

Lemon wedges for serving

Preheat the grill to medium-high heat.

Cook the quinoa according to package instructions.

Preheat the oven to 400°F (200°C). In a large bowl, toss the mixed vegetables with the olive oil. Season with salt and pepper. Spread the seasoned vegetables on a baking sheet and roast for 15 to 20 minutes.

Season the salmon fillets with salt and pepper. Grill for 4 to 5 minutes on each side, or until cooked through.

Divide the vegetables and quinoa among four plates or bowls. Top each with 1 salmon fillet. Squeeze lemon wedges over the top before serving.

Nutritional Info (per serving): *Calories: 380; Protein: 28g; Carbohydrates: 25g; Fat: 18g Fiber: 5g*

VEGGIE STIR-FRY WITH TOFU

SERVES 4

1 tablespoon sesame oil

2 cloves garlic, minced

1 teaspoon minced ginger

1 block tofu, pressed and cubed

2 cups sliced mixed vegetables (such as broccoli, carrots, and snap peas)

2 tablespoons soy sauce

Cooked brown rice for serving

Heat the sesame oil in a large skillet over medium heat. Add the garlic and ginger, cook for 1 minute, until fragrant, then set aside.

Add the tofu cubes to the skillet and cook until golden brown on all sides.

Add the mixed vegetables and soy sauce to the skillet. Stir-fry until the vegetables are tender-crisp.

Add the garlic and ginger to the skillet and mix well.

Serve the stir-fry in bowls over cooked brown rice.

Nutritional Info (per serving): *Calories: 280; Protein: 18g; Carbohydrates: 25g; Fiber: 6g Fat: 12g*

QUINOA-STUFFED BELL PEPPERS

SERVES 4

1 cup uncooked quinoa

1 (15-ounce) can black beans, rinsed and drained

1 cup corn kernels

1 cup diced tomatoes

1 teaspoon ground cumin

1 teaspoon chili powder

Salt and pepper to taste

4 bell peppers, tops cut and seeds and veins removed

½ cup shredded cheddar cheese (optional)

Preheat the oven to 375°F (190°C).

Cook the quinoa according to package instructions. Let cool.

In a large bowl, combine the cooked quinoa, black beans, corn, tomatoes, cumin, and chili powder. Season with salt and pepper.

Place the prepared peppers in a baking dish. Stuff each bell pepper with a quarter of the quinoa mixture.

Cover the stuffed peppers with foil and bake for 25 to 30 minutes.

If using cheese, sprinkle the cheese over the stuffed peppers and bake for an additional 5 minutes, or until the cheese is melted.

Nutritional Info (per serving without cheese): *Calories: 320; Protein: 12g; Carbohydrates: 60g; Fat: 4g; Fiber: 12g*

CHICKEN AND VEGETABLE QUINOA BOWL

SERVES 4

1 cup uncooked quinoa

4 tablespoons extra-virgin olive oil

2 boneless, skinless chicken breasts

Salt and pepper to taste

1 teaspoon Italian seasoning

2 cups sliced mixed vegetables (such as bell peppers, broccoli, and carrots)

2 tablespoons balsamic vinegar

Cook the quinoa according to package instructions. Let cool.

In a large skillet, heat 1 tablespoon of the olive oil over medium heat until it's shimmering.

Season the chicken breasts on both sides with salt, pepper, and the Italian seasoning. Place the chicken in the skillet and cook for 6 to 8 minutes per side. Remove the chicken from the skillet to a cutting board and slice into strips.

Clean the skillet, then heat 1 tablespoon of the olive oil over medium heat. Add the mixed vegetables and sauté until tender.

In a small bowl, whisk together the balsamic vinegar and the remaining 2 tablespoons olive oil to make the dressing.

Assemble four bowls with cooked quinoa, sliced chicken, and sautéed vegetables, and drizzle with the balsamic dressing.

Nutritional Info (per serving): *Calories: 380; Protein: 28g; Carbohydrates: 30g; Fat: 16g; Fiber: 5g*

LENTIL AND VEGETABLE SOUP

SERVES 6

1 tablespoon extra-virgin olive oil

1 onion, diced

2 carrots, diced

2 stalks celery, diced

2 cloves garlic, minced

1 cup dry lentils, sorted and rinsed

1 (14-ounce) can diced tomatoes

6 cups vegetable broth

1 teaspoon ground cumin

1 teaspoon paprika

Salt and pepper to taste

Fresh parsley for garnish

In a large stockpot, heat the olive oil until shimmering.

Add the onion, carrots, and celery and sauté until softened, about 5 minutes.

Add the garlic and cook for about 1 minute.

Add the lentils, diced tomatoes, vegetable broth, cumin, paprika, salt, and pepper to the pot.

Bring the soup to a boil, then reduce the heat and simmer for 25 to 30 minutes, or until the lentils are tender.

Serve hot, garnished with fresh parsley.

Nutritional Info (per serving): *Calories: 240; Protein: 14g; Carbohydrates: 40g; Fat: 2g; Fiber: 12g; Fat: 2g*

BAKED CHICKEN BREAST WITH SWEET POTATO AND ASPARAGUS

SERVES 4

4 boneless, skinless chicken breasts

2 tablespoons extra-virgin olive oil, plus more for drizzling

2 cloves garlic, minced

1 teaspoon paprika

Salt and pepper to taste

2 large sweet potatoes, peeled and cubed

1 bunch asparagus, trimmed

Fresh parsley for garnish

Preheat the oven to 400°F (200°C).

Place a small amount of oil in a baking dish then add the chicken breasts. Rub the chicken with the olive oil, garlic, and paprika. Season with salt and pepper.

Arrange the sweet potato cubes and asparagus around the chicken in the baking dish. Drizzle with additional olive oil and sprinkle the sweet potatoes and asparagus with salt and pepper.

Bake for 25 to 30 minutes, or until the chicken is cooked through and the vegetables are tender.

Garnish with fresh parsley before serving.

Nutritional Info (per serving): *Calories: 320; Protein: 30g; Carbohydrates: 25g; Fat: 12g; Fiber: 6g*

SHRIMP AND VEGETABLE STIR-FRY WITH BROWN RICE

SERVES 4

2 tablespoons soy sauce

1 tablespoon honey

1 tablespoon sesame oil

2 cloves garlic, minced

1 teaspoon minced ginger

1 tablespoon extra-virgin olive oil

1 pound shrimp, peeled and deveined

2 cups sliced mixed vegetables (such as bell peppers, broccoli, and snap peas)

Cooked brown rice for serving

In a small bowl, whisk together the soy sauce, honey, sesame oil, garlic, and ginger to make the sauce.

Heat the olive oil in a large skillet over medium-high heat. Add the shrimp and cook until pink and opaque, 2 to 3 minutes per side. Remove the shrimp from the skillet and set aside.

In the same skillet, add the mixed vegetables and stir-fry until tender-crisp.

Return the cooked shrimp to the skillet and pour the sauce over the shrimp and vegetables. Cook for an additional 2 to 3 minutes.

Serve the stir-fry in bowls over cooked brown rice.

Nutritional Info (per serving): *Calories: 280; Protein: 25g; Carbohydrates: 30g; Fat: 7g; Fiber: 5g*

TURKEY AND BLACK BEAN LETTUCE WRAPS

SERVES 4

1 tablespoon cooking oil

1 pound ground turkey

2 cloves garlic, minced

1 bell pepper, diced

1 teaspoon chili powder

1 teaspoon ground cumin

Salt and pepper to taste

1 (15-ounce) can black beans, rinsed and drained

1 cup corn kernels

Butter lettuce leaves for wrapping

Optional toppings: diced tomatoes, avocado slices, shredded cheese

In a large skillet over medium heat, heat the oil and cook the turkey, stirring often to break up the meat, until browned and cooked through, 5 to 7 minutes.

If there is a lot of residual oil in the skillet, remove it. Then add the garlic, bell pepper, chili powder, cumin, salt, and pepper. Stir to incorporate and cook for an additional 2 to 3 minutes.

Stir in the black beans and corn kernels. Cook until heated through.

Place a butter lettuce leaf on each of four plates.

Spoon a quarter of the turkey and black bean mixture onto each of the butter lettuce leaves.

Serve with optional toppings such as diced tomatoes, avocado slices, and shredded cheese.

Nutritional Info (per serving without toppings): *Calories: 280; Protein: 25g; Carbohydrates: 25g; Fat: 9g; Fiber: 8g*

BAKED COD WITH LEMON AND HERBS

SERVES 4

2 tablespoons extra-virgin olive oil, plus more for oiling the dish

4 cod fillets

2 tablespoons freshly squeezed lemon juice

2 cloves garlic, minced

1 teaspoon dried thyme

1 teaspoon dried oregano

Salt and pepper to taste

Lemon slices for serving

Preheat the oven to 400°F (200°C).

Lightly oil the bottom of a baking dish, then place the cod fillets in the dish. Drizzle the fillets with the olive oil and lemon juice.

Sprinkle the garlic, thyme, oregano, salt, and pepper over the cod fillets.

Bake for 15 to 20 minutes, or until the fish is opaque and flakes easily with a fork.

Garnish with lemon slices before serving.

Nutritional Info (per serving): *Calories: 180; Protein: 25g; Carbohydrates: 2g; Fat: 8g: Fiber: 0g*

VEGETABLE AND CHICKPEA CURRY WITH BROWN RICE

SERVES 4

1 tablespoon extra-virgin olive oil

1 onion, diced

2 cloves garlic, minced

1 tablespoon curry powder

1 teaspoon ground cumin

1 teaspoon ground coriander

1 (15-ounce) can chickpeas, rinsed and drained

1 (14-ounce) can diced tomatoes

2 cups sliced mixed vegetables (such as cauliflower, carrots, and peas)

1 (13.5-ounce) can coconut milk

Cooked brown rice for serving

Fresh cilantro for garnish

Heat the olive oil in a large stockpot over medium heat. The oil is ready when it's shimmering.

Add the onion and cook until softened, about 5 minutes.

Add the garlic and cook for about 1 minute.

Stir in the curry powder, cumin, and coriander. Cook for 1 minute, until fragrant.

Add the chickpeas, diced tomatoes, mixed vegetables, and coconut milk to the pot. Bring to a simmer and cook for 15 to 20 minutes, or until the vegetables are tender.

Prepare four bowls with cooked brown rice for serving.

Spoon the vegetable and chickpea curry over the brown rice.

Garnish with fresh cilantro before serving.

Nutritional Info (per serving without rice): *Calories: 320; Protein: 10g; Carbohydrates: 25g; Fat: 22g; Fiber: 8g*

LENTIL AND SPINACH-STUFFED PORTOBELLO MUSHROOMS

SERVES 4

4 large portobello mushrooms, stems removed

1 cup dry green lentils, sorted and rinsed

2 cups vegetable broth

1 tablespoon extra-virgin olive oil

1 onion, diced

2 cups chopped fresh spinach

2 cloves garlic, minced

1 teaspoon dried thyme

Salt and pepper to taste

¼ cup grated Parmesan cheese (optional)

Preheat the oven to 375°F (190°C). Line a baking sheet with parchment paper.

Place the portobello mushrooms on the prepared baking sheet, gill side up. Set aside.

In a medium saucepan, combine the lentils and vegetable broth. Bring to a boil, then reduce the heat and simmer for 20 to 25 minutes, or until the lentils are tender and the liquid is absorbed.

In a skillet, heat the olive oil over medium heat. Add the onion and cook until softened, about 5 minutes.

Add the spinach to the skillet and cook until wilted, about 1 minute.

Add the garlic and cook for about 1 more minute.

Stir the cooked lentils into the skillet with the spinach and onion mixture. Season with the thyme, salt, and pepper.

Spoon the lentil and spinach mixture into each portobello mushroom cap, pressing down gently.

If using, sprinkle the Parmesan cheese over the stuffed mushrooms.

Bake for 15 to 20 minutes, or until the mushrooms are tender and the cheese is melted.

Serve hot as a main dish or alongside a salad for a complete meal.

Nutritional Info (per serving without the Parmesan cheese): *Calories: 240; Protein: 14g; Carbohydrates: 38g; Fat: 4g; Fiber: 15g*

6

YOUR TOP 7 PHYSICAL FITNESS TESTS

Aging doesn't mean we must simply resign ourselves to an inevitable physical demise. Yes, the constant wear and tear on our bodies will take a toll, but how much of a toll it takes is largely in our control. It's important to keep tabs on where we are in life in our physical journey. The expression "use it or lose it" couldn't be truer than when it applies to our body's physicality and functionality. Our balance, strength, flexibility, endurance, and cardiorespiratory fitness will diminish greatly as we age, but the rate of decline can be slowed tremendously if we are aware earlier that we are falling behind the norm for our age. These easy at-home tests will help you assess where you stack up to others your age. If your results are not as good as you would like, this can give you an indication of what you need to work on and can serve as an inspiration for you to take the necessary steps to improve in those areas that are lacking or deficient. A regular exercise program involving strength training, stretching, and cardiovascular exercises can increase your conditioning such that you're able to physically perform within the expected range of your age group.

To see a video of how these tests should be performed, use this QR code:

SINGLE-LEG BALANCE TEST

As we get older, our posture and balance change and often not for the better. Muscles tend to weaken and there are neurological changes that can affect our balance. The Single-Leg Balance Test is used to assess posture and balance control while standing still. Clinicians often use this test to help diagnose and assess certain conditions, such as neurological problems (peripheral neuropathy—nerve damage to the legs, Parkinson's disease, cervical spondylosis), vestibular problems (inner ear abnormalities), and intermittent claudication (lower-extremity skeletal muscle pain that occurs during exercise).

Instructions

1. Stand upright near a wall or close to a sturdy object that can steady you in the event you lose your balance.
2. Place your hands on the sides of your hips and raise one foot off the ground at least 1 foot. Hold your foot in the air as long as you can without taking your hands off your hips and without letting your foot touch the ground. Once either of these happens, the test is over.
3. Record your time.
4. Repeat the same balance challenge, but this time with your eyes closed. Record this time.
5. Compare your two times (eyes open and eyes closed) with the data in the tables on the next page.

SINGLE-LEG BALANCE TEST: WOMEN

AGE	EYES OPEN	EYES CLOSED
18 to 39 years	43 seconds	9 seconds
40 to 49 years	40 seconds	7 seconds
50 to 59 years	36 seconds	5 seconds
60 to 69 years	25 seconds	3 seconds
70 to 79 years	11 seconds	2 seconds
80 to 99 years	7 seconds	1 second

Source: Adapted from Journal of Geriatric Physical Therapy *Vol. 30;1:07*

SINGLE-LEG BALANCE TEST: MEN

AGE	EYES OPEN	EYES CLOSED
18 to 39 years	43 seconds	10 seconds
40 to 49 years	40 seconds	7 seconds
50 to 59 years	38 seconds	5 seconds
60 to 69 years	29 seconds	3 seconds
70 to 79 years	18 seconds	2 seconds
80 to 99 years	6 seconds	1 second

Source: Adapted from Journal of Geriatric Physical Therapy *Vol. 30;1:07*

PUSH-UP TEST

This test measures your upper-body muscular strength and endurance. Three critical muscle groups are used: the chest (pectoralis muscles), the back of the upper arm (triceps muscles), and the shoulders (anterior and medial deltoids). When performing a full, classic push-up, you are lifting approximately 75 percent of your total body weight. When using a modified push-up position (recommended for women in this test) with the knees and lower legs on the ground, you lift approximately 60 percent of your weight.

Instructions

1. Start in the standard "down" position (fingers pointed forward on the ground, hands separated a little wider than the shoulders, back straight, head up, toes are used as the pivot point). If you can't complete a push-up this way, use a modified knee push-up (knees are the pivot point and are in contact with the floor, the feet are spread comfortably apart with the soles of the feet facing upward).

2. Raise your body by straightening your elbows, then once you are all the way up and your elbows have reached a full straightened position, lower your body back into the "down" position until your chin touches or almost touches the floor. The stomach should not come into contact with the floor.

3. Keep your back straight at all times through the exercise, and when going to the top of the push-up, your arms must be in a fully straight position, but don't lock your elbows.

4. Do as many push-ups as you can until full exhaustion (unable to complete a repetition or failure to maintain proper technique for two consecutive repetitions). Record the final number of completed push-ups and compare it to the data in the charts below and on the next page.

PUSH-UP TEST: WOMEN

	30 TO 39 YEARS OLD	40 TO 49 YEARS OLD	50 TO 59 YEARS OLD	60+ YEARS OLD
Excellent	27 or more	24 or more	21 or more	14 or more
Very Good	20 to 26	15 to 23	11 to 20	12 to 16
Good	13 to 19	11 to 14	7 to 10	5 to 11
Fair	8 to 12	5 to 10	2 to 6	2 to 4
Needs Improvement	7 or less	4 or less	1 or less	1 or less

Source: Adapted from American Council on Exercise

PUSH-UP TEST: MEN

	30 TO 39 YEARS OLD	40 TO 49 YEARS OLD	50 TO 59 YEARS OLD	60+ YEARS OLD
Excellent	30 or more	25 or more	21 or more	18 or more
Very Good	22 to 29	17 to 24	13 to 20	11 to 17
Good	17 to 21	13 to 16	10 to 12	8 to 10
Fair	12 to 16	10 to 12	7 to 9	5 to 7
Needs Improvement	11 or less	9 or less	6 or less	4 or less

Source: Adapted from American Council on Exercise

SIT-AND-REACH TEST

This test is an indirect measure of hamstring, hip, and lower-back flexibility. As we get older, our soft tissues become more rigid and less elastic, contributing to a loss of flexibility. There are a few variations of this test, the most common being one that utilizes a specially designed sit-and-reach box. Most people don't have access to this box, so the version included here is one that only requires a tape measure or yardstick and another person to assist in the measurement.

Instructions

1. Find an open space on the floor and place a yardstick down. Hold the yardstick down with a piece of tape at the 15-inch mark.
2. Sit on the ground with your legs extended and open into a V. The yardstick should be between your legs. Place the soles of your feet so that they're even with the 15-inch mark on the yardstick.
3. Clasp your hands together in front of you, one on top of the other, then have someone hold your knees down so that

your legs stay flat on the ground while you slowly reach forward as far as you can along the yardstick.

4. Exhale as you're reaching forward, and when you reach as far as you can, hold it for at least 1 second, and record the distance that you reach.

5. Repeat the reach two more times, recording each distance. Choose the best of the three reaches and compare it to the data in the chart below.

SIT-AND-REACH TEST: GOOD FLEXIBILITY RESULTS

AGE	WOMEN: FARTHEST REACH	MEN: FARTHEST REACH
25 years	21.5 inches	19.5 inches
35 years	20.5 inches	18.5 inches
45 years	20 inches	17.5 inches
55 years	19 inches	16.5 inches
65 years	17.5 inches	15.5 inches

Source: Mayo Clinic

Cardiovascular fitness is your body's ability to use oxygen to produce energy while you're engaging in physical activity. It uses three large systems in coordination to allow you to carry out the task at hand, whether it be running, walking, cycling, or hiking. Your cardiovascular system (heart and blood vessels), respiratory system (lungs), and musculoskeletal system (muscles) work together during physical exertion. If one or more of these systems is impaired or not up to par, then your ability to carry out physical activity without enduring great stress or your ability to recover from said activity can be extremely challenging. Your cardiovascular fitness is not just important for completing simple tasks such as climbing steps or getting from the security line to your gate at the airport without getting winded, but it also speaks volumes about your health and what your potential health outcomes might be. The following tests will help you assess your cardiovascular fitness.

1.5-MILE WALK/RUN

This test is designed to assess cardiovascular fitness by challenging the body to endure prolonged exercise. Our heart, lungs, and muscles must work together when we are engaged in an aerobic activity such as walking, running, jumping, and squatting. These movements are fundamental not just in many sports but in completing our daily life functions. When you're walking down the aisle in the grocery store and you stop and bend down to take a closer look at something on the bottom shelf, you need some level of cardiovascular fitness as well as leg strength and balance. If you're too sedentary, your fitness level starts to decline, and your performance ability goes along with it. This test will give you a sense of your cardiovascular fitness condition. If the results show a need for improvement, hopefully you will be inspired to make the necessary lifestyle changes.

Instructions

1. Find a location that will allow you to walk or run for 1.5 miles without interruption. This can be a park, track, sidewalk, safe road, or wherever there is a surface that will let you move unimpeded. If you use a treadmill, set it to a 1 percent incline to better simulate outdoor conditions.
2. Complete the 1.5 miles as fast as you can, whether it's running or walking or a combination of the two.

1.5-MILE RUN/WALK

PERCENTILE	30 TO 39 YEARS OLD		40 TO 49 YEARS OLD		50 TO 59 YEARS OLD		60 TO 69 YEARS OLD	
	Men	Women	Men	Women	Men	Women	Men	Women
90	9:52	11:43	10:09	12:25	11:09	13:58	12:10	15:32
80	10:38	12:53	11:09	13:38	12:08	15:14	13:25	16:46
70	11:09	13:41	11:52	14:33	12:53	16:26	14:33	18:05
60	11:49	14:33	12:25	15:17	13:53	17:19	15:20	18:52
50	12:25	15:14	13:05	16:13	14:33	18:05	16:19	20:08
40	12:53	15:56	13:50	17:11	15:14	19:10	17:19	20:55
30	13:48	16:46	14:33	18:26	16:16	20:17	18:39	22:34
20	14:33	18:18	15:32	19:43	17:30	21:57	20:13	23:55
10	15:56	20:13	17:04	21:52	19:24	23:55	23:27	26:32

Adapted from the Cooper Institute and HumanKinetics.com

Dr. Ian's Tip

PUMP WEIGHTS

The idea that lifting weights is only for sweaty muscular men in noisy gyms is not only arcane but misleading and costly. Everyone at every age should engage in some type of resistance training that puts demands on your muscles and other soft tissues. The benefits of strength training are enormous. Improved insulin sensitivity, lowered blood pressure, improved flexibility and balance, fat burning, and increased metabolic rate are just some of the health benefits to be gained. If you don't have bands or weights to use, no problem. Do exercises using your own body weight (push-ups, pull-ups, squats, etc.). They, too, can be very effective.

YMCA 3-MINUTE SUBMAXIMAL STEP TEST

This test assesses your fitness level based on how quickly your heart rate recovers after strenuous exercise.

Instructions

1. Use a 12-inch step (either a staircase, platform box, or step stool) and complete 24 steps per minute for 3 minutes. Step up on the platform with the first foot. Bring the second foot up on the platform. Lower the first foot back to the ground. Lower the second foot back to the ground to your start position. When both feet are back on the ground, that is considered to be 1 complete step.

2. Within 5 seconds of completing the steps, measure your resting heart rate for 60 seconds. This number is your recovery pulse. You can measure this using your index and middle finger on the inside of your wrist at the base of your thumb.

3. Using the tables on the next page, find your age range and recovery pulse, then see what category of fitness you fall under.

RATINGS FOR WOMEN, BASED ON AGE

	18 TO 25 YEARS	26 TO 35 YEARS	36 TO 45 YEARS	46 TO 55 YEARS	56 TO 65 YEARS	65+ YEARS
Excellent	52–81	58–80	51–84	63–91	60–92	70–92
Good	85–93	85–92	89–96	95–101	97–103	96–101
Above Average	96–102	95–101	100–104	104–110	106–111	104–111
Average	104–110	104–110	107–112	113–118	113–118	116–121
Below Average	113–120	113–119	115–120	120–124	119–127	123–126
Poor	122–131	122–129	124–132	126–132	129–135	128–133
Very Poor	135–169	134–171	137–169	137–171	141–174	135–155

RATINGS FOR MEN, BASED ON AGE

	18 TO 25 YEARS	26 TO 35 YEARS	36 TO 45 YEARS	46 TO 55 YEARS	56 TO 65 YEARS	65+ YEARS
Excellent	50–76	51–76	49–76	56–82	60–77	59–81
Good	79–84	79–85	80–88	87–93	86–94	87–92
Above Average	88–93	88–94	88–92	95–101	97–100	94–102
Average	95–100	96–102	100–105	103–111	103–109	104–110
Below Average	102–107	104–110	108–113	113–119	111–117	114–118
Poor	111–119	114–121	116–124	121–126	119–128	121–126
Very Poor	124–157	126–161	130–163	131–159	131–154	130–151

SIT-UP (CURL-UP) TEST

This test is used to measure abdominal strength and endurance. Instead of doing a full sit-up, you will be doing what's called a curl-up, which is about half of a full sit-up. This modified version is being used because it's much safer for the exerciser (it avoids lower-back and neck strain), and it's a more reliable indicator of abdominal strength and endurance because it doesn't use the recruitment of other muscles; rather, it specifically focuses on the abdominal muscles. If you suffer from lower-back or neck pain, be careful if you decide to perform this test.

Instructions

1. Start in the "down" position with your back on the ground and your arms folded across your chest. Your feet should be flat on the floor and both knees bent at a 90-degree angle.
2. Curl up by lifting your shoulder blades off the ground toward your knees. You don't have to go all the way up to your knees, rather about halfway there (30 degrees of trunk flexion).
3. Lower your torso back down until your shoulders touch the ground. (Your head does not need to touch the ground.)
4. Exhale on the way up and inhale on the way down.
5. Complete as many curl-ups as you can, with proper form of feet staying on the ground and knees bent, until you are totally exhausted and can't do anymore. Record this final number and compare it to those on the chart below.

1-MINUTE SIT-UP TEST: WOMEN

	26 TO 35 YEARS OLD	36 TO 45 YEARS OLD	46 TO 55 YEARS OLD	56 TO 65 YEARS OLD	66+ YEARS OLD
Excellent	54–70	54–74	48–73	44–63	34–54
Good	44–50	42–48	37–44	35–42	31–33
Above Average	37–41	35–38	33–36	27–32	26–29
Average	33–36	30–32	30–32	23–25	21–25
Below Average	28–32	23–28	25–28	18–22	16–20
Poor	22–26	19–22	19–23	11–15	10–13
Very Poor	7–20	4–16	2–13	1–8	0–9

Source: Adapted from the American Council on Exercise

1-MINUTE SIT-UP TEST: MEN

	26 TO 35 YEARS OLD	36 TO 45 YEARS OLD	46 TO 55 YEARS OLD	56 TO 65 YEARS OLD	66+ YEARS OLD
Excellent	62–80	60–79	61–78	56–77	50–66
Good	53–58	48–57	52–57	48–53	38–44
Above Average	44–52	43–45	44–51	41–46-22	31–35
Average	37–41	33–39	36–41	33–39	26–30
Below Average	33–36	29–32	29–33	28–32	22–24
Poor	26–32	24–28	21–25	21–25	15–21
Very Poor	7–21	6–21	6–16	5–20	5–12

Source: Adapted from the American Council on Exercise

SQUAT TEST

This test is a good measure of your lower-body strength and muscular endurance. When done properly, this exercise will work your quads, glutes, calves, and core. This is not a timed test, rather one that works by doing the exercise until exhaustion and your form breaks down.

Instructions

1. Stand with your feet just a little wider than your shoulders and your toes pointing just slightly outward at an angle.
2. Keep your head facing forward in a neutral position aligned with your back. Keep your back straight.
3. As you lower your body into the squat position, bend your knees and keep lowering your body until your knees are at a 90-degree bend and your thighs are parallel to the ground (like sitting in a chair). As you are lowering your body, lift and extend your hands out and forward until they are parallel to the ground.

4. Throughout the exercise, keep your back straight, shoulders back, chest forward, arms extended out, and feet planted on the ground.

5. When your thighs are parallel to the ground, return to the standing position by pushing with your feet, legs, and hips and thrusting upward.

6. Continue to do the squats until your mechanics break down and you're unable to do two consecutive squats with proper form. Record that number and compare it to the date in the tables below.

SQUAT TEST FOR WOMEN

	30 TO 39	40 TO 49	50 TO 59	60+
Excellent	More than 26	More than 23	More than 20	More than 17
Good	24–26	21–23	18–20	15–17
Above Average	21–23	18–20	15–17	12–14
Average	18–20	15–17	12–14	9–11
Below Average	15–17	12–14	9–11	6–8
Poor	12–14	9–11	6–8	3–5
Very Poor	Less than 12	Less than 9	Less than 6	Less than 3

SQUAT TEST FOR MEN

	30 TO 39	40 TO 49	50 TO 59	60+
Excellent	More than 32	More than 29	More than 26	More than 23
Good	30–32	27–29	24–26	21–23
Above Average	27–29	24–26	21–23	18–20
Average	24–26	21–23	18–20	15–17
Below Average	21–23	18–20	15–17	12–14
Poor	18–20	15–17	12–14	9–11
Very Poor	Less than 18	Less than 15	Less than 12	Less than 9

Source: Australian College of Sports & Fitness

VERTICAL JUMP ASSESSMENT

The purpose of this test is to evaluate your standing vertical jump height. This maneuver requires good lower-body muscle strength as well as flexibility and coordination. The American Council on Exercise has published how this assessment is to be performed. You will need a flat, stable floor that provides good traction, a smooth wall with a relatively high ceiling, a measuring tape or stick, a step stool or small ladder, and chalk that's a different color than the wall.

Instructions

1. Stand adjacent to a wall, with the inside shoulder of the dominant arm approximately 6 inches (15 cm) from the wall.
2. Rub chalk onto your index finger, then mark your standing height against the wall with chalk. This is the mark that will be used when comparing to the maximal height achieved on a vertical jump.
3. Lower your arms and, without any pause or step, drop into a squat movement before exploding upward into a vertical jump, jumping as high as you can. Good form is important in achieving the highest jump, so make sure to use your arms and legs to create maximal explosive effort.
4. When you reach the highest point, touch the wall and create a mark with the chalk.
5. Measure the vertical distance between the starting height mark and the new chalk mark.
6. Repeat the jump three times and use the maximal height achieved for the final assessment.

WOMEN NORMS FOR VERTICAL JUMP ASSESSMENT (CM)

AGE (YEARS)	EXCELLENT	VERY GOOD	GOOD	FAIR	NEEDS IMPROVEMENT
30–39	>36	32–35	28–31	24–27	≤23
40–49	>31	27–30	23–26	18–22	≤17
50–59	>25	21–24	16–20	10–15	≤9
60–69	>19	15–18	11–14	10–15	≤6

MEN NORMS FOR VERTICAL JUMP ASSESSMENT (CM)

AGE (YEARS)	EXCELLENT	VERY GOOD	GOOD	FAIR	NEEDS IMPROVEMENT
30–39	>52	46–51	40–45	31–39	≤30
40–49	>43	36–42	32–35	26–31	≤25
50–59	>41	34–40	28–33	18–27	≤17
60–69	>33	29–32	25–28	18–24	≤17

Adapted from Gibson, A.L., Wagner, D.R., & Heyward, V.H. (2019). Advanced Fitness Assessment and Exercise Prescription (8th ed.). Champaign, Ill.: Human Kinetics, 175.

The Inspiration

Marcus is an overweight 62-year-old man who leads a relatively sedentary lifestyle because of his desk job as a trucking company dispatcher and his lack of regular physical activity. Recently, he had been experiencing fatigue, shortness of breath, and general feelings of sluggishness. His typical day involves long hours spent sitting at his desk, followed by evenings relaxing on the couch. He rarely engages in structured exercise and has noticed a decline in his overall energy levels and physical stamina over the years but has largely ignored the warning signs of his declining physical fitness. However, two weeks ago, a close friend of his was walking up his stairs to go to bed after dinner and fell to the ground with an excruciating pain in his chest and shortness of breath. He was rushed to the hospital and diagnosed as having a heart attack. Fortunately, he survived, but needed immediate surgery to clear the blockage in two blood vessels that feed his heart.

The Plan

The very next day, Marcus was finally motivated to change, so he decided to perform a couple of at-home fitness tests to gauge his current fitness level. He started with a simple walking test, measuring how far he can walk in 10 minutes. To his dismay, he found himself winded and fatigued after just a short distance.

Marcus then attempted a basic strength test, doing as many push-ups as he could in 1 minute. Struggling to complete even a few, he realized the extent of his muscular weakness and lack of upper-body strength.

Upon completing these fitness tests, Marcus was faced with the reality of his current physical condition. He acknowledged that his sedentary lifestyle had taken a toll on his health and quality of life. However, rather than feeling discouraged, Marcus saw this as an opportunity to make positive changes and improve his overall well-being.

With a newfound determination and fear of suffering a similar fate as his friend, Marcus set specific, achievable goals for himself. He aimed to increase his walking distance by at least 50 percent within the next month and to gradually build up his strength to perform 10 consecutive push-ups. He recognized the importance of incorporating regular exercise into his daily routine, so he decided to start by incorporating short walks into his day, gradually increasing both the duration and intensity over time. Additionally, he committed to incorporating strength training exercises into his weekly routine, focusing on bodyweight exercises and resistance bands to lose weight, build muscle, and improve his overall strength.

The Change

Over the following weeks, Marcus diligently followed his exercise plan, gradually increased his walking distance, regularly got up from his desk at work to take physical activity breaks, and improved his strength through regular workouts. He also made small changes to his diet, emphasizing whole, nutritious foods and staying hydrated. Through self-assessment, goal-setting, and consistent effort, Marcus successfully improves his fitness levels and overall health. By taking proactive steps to test his level of fitness then address his sedentary lifestyle, he not only increased his physical stamina and strength but also experienced improved mood, energy levels, and overall wellbeing. He is committed to testing himself regularly to help monitor his fitness journey.

7

YOUR TOP EXERCISES

Exercise is extremely important not just for your physical health but for your mental health as well. Exercise provides physical challenges that your body needs to keep functioning properly from your muscles all the way down to your organs. The saying "If you don't use it, you lose it" is quite appropriate when it comes to describing the importance of regular exercise and the impact it has on growing and maintaining your body's physicality and functioning. Think of the human body like a complicated sports car. When you don't drive a sports car enough or maintain it properly, it starts to break down from underuse. It needs to be driven at different speeds to keep all the mechanical systems operating efficiently and effectively. The same is needed for our body. There are hundreds of different exercises that can be performed inside or outside of a gym. Which exercises are best for you will depend on numerous variables. Your goals, equipment availability, medical conditions, and conditioning level are all different from person to person. You might be trying to put on more muscle, while someone else is satisfied with their muscle volume but wants to improve their flexibility. Two of the most important factors in your making progress toward your goals are choosing the right type of exercises and being consistent in what you choose. Also, check with your healthcare provider before starting any fitness program to make sure it's safe and compatible with your health needs and abilities.

The way this chapter works is quite simple. The exercises listed in your decade should not be considered the *only* exercises you should do, rather they are suggestions of what could have the greatest impact. You should try to discover and learn other exercises that might also be beneficial. After you learn the best exercises for your decade, there is a plan that incorporates four major movements that are essential for all of us, regardless of our age or goals. These movements are fundamental to how you live and the activities you perform in daily life, whether it's picking up groceries or climbing the stairs at night to get to the bedroom. Of course, look at your decade's suggestions first, but don't stop there. Look at the others as well, and by all means try adding some of those exercises to expand your regimen. With so many exercises and workouts available to you, there are seemingly infinite combinations of movements and modifications that can be performed to keep things fresh and engaging. There is not one workout plan that is the best. The beauty of having so many exercise options is that you can customize your workout whether you're in a gym or at home or a simple fitness studio. Don't be afraid to safely experiment with exercises you've never done before or that might challenge you. You will eventually find a groove that makes physical activity a staple in your life, and that will pay dividends not only now but for years to come.

30S

This is a busy decade with so many life changes and challenges. Starting a family, building a career, and maintaining a robust social life are just a few of the obligations that can come with this decade. But this is also the time where you will have reached many physical peaks such as bone mass, muscle mass, and flexibility. The physical decline begins during these years but can be slowed or stalled if you undertake a regular fitness routine. A lot is going to happen to your body during your 30s. Your fast-twitch muscle fibers, which are responsible for explosive movements, are the first to decline as you age, but this can be counteracted with high-intensity interval training (HIIT), a type of exercise in which the exertion alternates between brief periods of high intensity followed by rest or low intensity, then the cycle is repeated. (Think about walking at a fast pace for 30 seconds, then walking slowly for 30 seconds, then returning to the fast pace and starting the cycle all over again.) Flexibility begins to decrease approximately 1 percent per year, which makes stretching and exercises like Pilates, yoga, and Tai Chi critical to keep you limber. These are the years where most women who plan to get pregnant will have children. This requires a certain level of physical strength not to just carry a baby in the womb, but bending down and picking up toddlers, running after them, and trying to match their boundless energy. Maintaining or increasing strength and improving endurance for both men and women is important and can be achieved with the right type and frequency of exercises.

This is a performance decade where you may be training for fitness competitions, specific sports, or mental well-being, as regular exercise has consistently shown to have a positive impact on a person's mental health. Vigorous exercise sessions involving cardio and strength training will help develop a strong heart and lungs, an important combination for physical endurance. This is also the easiest time to build good muscle mass that will serve you not only now but for many decades to come. As you plan your exercise schedule, remember that you're not just seeking improvements for now, but you're making an important investment in your future.

40S

This is a critical decade for you to maintain or build muscle. Soft tissues become more rigid and less pliable as we age, so it's also important to improve your flexibility. After years of putting lots of stress on your joints, early signs of joint problems might appear during your 40s. Committing to a regular exercise regimen that includes important body motions will go a long way in delaying the onset of joint issues and other chronic conditions that begin to appear in this decade.

Adding recreational sports to your exercise regimen is a great way to still get in the various body movements without subjecting your body to extreme amounts of resistance, which can become increasingly difficult to endure well as we age. A nice 30- to 45-minute bike ride in which you climb some hills or change up your speed throughout different segments of the ride can be a great way to work on your lower-body muscles as well as your cardiovascular endurance. Playing tennis or pickleball can be helpful in working on your balance, agility, eye-hand coordination, and improving your cardiovascular fitness.

50s

Your body has changed in many ways from what it looked and felt like when you were in your 20s, 30s, and 40s. Your reflexes might be a tad slower, your muscles don't have the same pop, your skin is not as tight, and your endurance doesn't measure up to what it used to be. Understanding that age inevitably takes a toll on all of us should be acknowledged but should not be considered an excuse to decrease your activity level and become passive. The attitude that "whatever's gonna happen is gonna happen" is one of resignation and acceptance. You can take a more positive and proactive approach to your aging. Your 50s still present a lot of opportunities to improve and grow and increase not just the length of your life but the quality as well. Make no mistake, these 10 years are critical as they can absolutely shape what the rest of your life will look and feel like.

When most people reach this age, they have lost a tremendous amount of muscle mass since their 20s and 30s. To make things even more undesirable, body fat percentage has likely gone up and that number staring back from the scale is not what it used to be. If these circumstances apply to you, understand that you are not alone. The good news, however, is that you can change things around in a relatively short period of time by not just eating better but by choosing the right exercises and being consistent in your workout routine frequency and intensity. This is a decade to really focus on building and maintaining muscle, protecting or improving your bone health, making sure the range of motion at your joints remains optimal, and keeping your balance/coordination performance at a high level to avoid dangerous falls.

60s+

Welcome to the decade where what you have and haven't done the last 59 years starts revealing itself. In our 60s, we experience a range of physical changes and life transitions. Physically, there can be a decrease in muscle mass and bone density, leading to increased risk of fractures and osteoporosis. Skin may become drier and less elastic, leading to wrinkles and age spots. Women can still be dealing with the aftereffects from the hormonal changes that occurred during menopause. Additionally, sensory changes such as declining vision and hearing may become more apparent. Life-wise, many individuals in their 60s may retire from their careers, leading to a shift in daily routines and social dynamics. Some may become grandparents (though for many this can happen even earlier), experiencing the joys of family expansion. Health management becomes increasingly important, with regular check-ups and screenings becoming routine. Overall, the 60s marks a stage of both physical changes and new life chapters that should be viewed as a series of wonderful beginnings and vast opportunities.

There are many different types of exercises that can be performed in this decade, whether cardio or strength training or postural training. With each passing decade of our life, our bodies change; so our physical/exercise needs change in order to keep our muscles, bones, brain, and soft tissues operating at their best. What you needed to challenge your body in your 20s can be very different from what you need in your 60s. Balance is typically not a concern for someone in their 30s, but it can be a major concern for those 60 and over. In the chart that follows, you will find the exercise classifications that will potentially give you the greatest benefit for your current decade of life. The chart also lists various types of exercises and the recommended frequency per week or the number of repetitions or sets you should do. Choose from this list and vary the exercises between workouts. You are not expected to do all the exercises in one session—rather, over the course of multiple sessions in any given week, try to do as many of them as you can. Choose the exercises that best suit the space and equipment that is available to you. For example, if you have only an empty fitness studio or hotel room with no equipment, choose a 20-minute round of HIIT using bodyweight exercises. If you're in a gym that is fully equipped with machines and free weights (dumbbells and barbells), choose exercises that take advantage of the equipment available, such as bench presses, biceps curls, deadlifts, and kettlebell swings.

Where the exercise calls for using weights or resistance bands, use a weight or resistance strength with which you can do a full 10 repetitions. If you are trying to increase your strength dramatically and quickly, your weight requirements and the style in which you lift will be different. If you have the means and opportunity, consult with a professional trainer to help you determine a program that works well for you. I have created a free fitness app that will show you exercises and programs you can do either at home or in the gym with and without equipment. Go to funfitnessbros.com and download the app for free.

For video explanations of how to do these exercises, scan this QR code:

AGE	EXERCISE CATEGORY	TIMES PER WEEK
30s	Cardio	3
	Compound Strength Training	1-2
	High Impact	2-3
	High-Intensity Interval Training (HIIT)	2-3
	Pilates	1
	Recreational Sports/Activities	2
	Strength Training	3
40s	Bodyweight	2
	Cardio	3
	Compound Exercises	1
	High Impact	1-2
	High-Intensity Interval Training (HIIT)	2
	Low Impact	1
	Recreational Sports/Activities	1-2
	Strength Training	2-3
	Stretching (Yoga or other exercises)	3
		1-2
50s	Balance Training	2
	Bodyweight	2
	Cardiovascular	2-3
	Core	Work in while doing other exercises
	High Impact	2
	High-Intensity Interval Training (HIIT)	1 (high impact)
	Recreational Sports/Activities	1 (high/low impact)
	Pilates (Alternate with Yoga)	1-2
	Strength Training	1
	Stretching	2-3
	Yoga (Alternate with Pilates)	1-2
60s+	Balance Training	2
	Cardiovascular	2-3
	Postural	1
	Recreational Sports/Activities	1-2
	Strength Training	2-3
	Stretching	3
	Yoga	1

Below is a brief description of the exercise categories. Read through them and decide which will work for you and will help you reach your fitness/physical goals. If possible, working even briefly with a fitness expert or personal trainer can be extremely helpful in getting you on the right track safely and productively. If this isn't possible, there are lots of excellent videos online that can help inform and guide you.

BALANCE TRAINING

Balance training is a type of workout that focuses on enhancing an individual's ability to maintain stability and equilibrium. It involves a variety of exercises and activities that challenge the body's balance mechanisms, including proprioception (the body's awareness of its position in space), coordination, and muscular strength. The primary goal of balance training is to improve the body's ability to control its center of gravity over its base of support, thereby reducing the risk of falls and enhancing overall physical performance. This type of training is particularly important for athletes, older adults, and individuals recovering from injury or surgery.

Balance training exercises can vary widely in complexity and intensity, ranging from simple static exercises like standing on one leg to more dynamic activities such as walking on a balance beam or using stability balls. Common tools used in balance training include balance boards, wobble boards, stability discs, and foam pads. By regularly engaging in balance training, individuals can improve their proprioception, which helps them better sense and respond to changes in their environment. This can translate to improved coordination, agility, and reaction time, all of which are essential for activities ranging from sports and fitness to everyday tasks like walking and climbing stairs.

Another important benefit of balance training is that it can help strengthen the muscles that support the joints, particularly those in the ankles, knees, and hips. Stronger muscles not only contribute to better balance but also reduce the risk of injury during physical activity. Stability and mobility are improved, and so is the confidence with which one moves.

The following are some balance training exercises:

- **Balance board exercises:** Use a balance board to perform various movements, such as squats or lunges, while keeping the board level.
- **BOSU ball exercises:** Use a half-dome stability ball to perform exercises like squats, lunges, or core work while maintaining balance on the unstable surface.
- **Single-leg balance:** Stand on one leg while maintaining stability and control. You can also hold dumbbells while doing this to give yourself a greater challenge.
- **Stability ball exercises:** Perform exercises like planks or push-ups while balancing on a stability ball.
- **Tai Chi:** This is a mind-body practice involving slow, deliberate movements and shifting weight from one leg to another, promoting balance and coordination.
- **Yoga poses:** Poses like Tree pose or Warrior 3 pose challenge balance and stability while improving strength and flexibility.

BODYWEIGHT TRAINING

Bodyweight training, also known as calisthenics, is a form of exercise that utilizes the body's own weight as resistance to build strength, endurance, flexibility, and overall fitness. Unlike traditional weight-lifting, which relies on external weights like dumbbells, kettlebells, or barbells, bodyweight exercises use movements that engage multiple muscle groups simultaneously.

One of the primary benefits of bodyweight training is its versatility and accessibility. It can be performed virtually anywhere, requiring minimal or no equipment. This makes it an ideal option for individuals who may not have access to a gym or prefer to exercise outdoors.

Bodyweight training also offers functional fitness benefits, as many of the movements mimic everyday activities and promote better movement patterns. Additionally, since the exercises engage multiple muscle groups simultaneously, they help improve overall coordination and balance.

Some common bodyweight exercises include push-ups, pull-ups, squats, lunges, planks, triceps dips, and burpees, among others. These exercises can be modified to accommodate different fitness levels, making them accessible to beginners and advanced athletes alike.

One of the advantages of bodyweight training beyond it being accessible to people of all fitness levels is that it can be easily customized to target specific muscle groups or fitness goals. Whether someone aims to build muscle, improve cardiovascular health, or increase flexibility, there are countless variations and progressions available to keep workouts challenging and effective.

CARDIO

Cardiovascular training, commonly known as cardio, encompasses various forms of physical activity that primarily aim to enhance the health and functionality of the cardiovascular system, which includes the heart, blood vessels, and lungs. The main objective of cardio training is to elevate the heart rate to a certain level for an extended period, thereby challenging the cardiovascular system and improving its efficiency.

Cardio exercises typically involve rhythmic, repetitive movements that engage large muscle groups and increase oxygen consumption. Examples of popular cardio exercises include running, cycling, swimming, brisk walking, jumping rope, and aerobic dance classes. These activities can be performed at different intensities, durations, and frequencies to achieve specific fitness goals, such as improving endurance, burning calories, or reducing the risk of cardiovascular diseases.

Engaging in regular cardio training offers numerous health benefits, including:

- **Improved heart health:** These exercises strengthen the heart muscle, making it more efficient at pumping blood throughout the body. This can help lower blood pressure and reduce the risk of heart disease and stroke.
- **Enhanced lung function:** Cardiovascular activities increase the demand for oxygen, which improves lung capacity and efficiency. Over time, this can lead to better respiratory function and increased endurance.
- **Weight management:** Cardio workouts burn calories and promote fat loss, making them an effective component of weight management and body composition improvement programs.
- **Increased endurance:** Regular cardio training improves stamina and endurance by enhancing the body's ability to deliver oxygen to working muscles and remove waste products, such as carbon dioxide and lactic acid.
- **Stress reduction:** Cardiovascular exercise triggers the release of endorphins, neurotransmitters that promote feelings of well-being and reduce stress and anxiety levels.
- **Better sleep:** Engaging in regular cardio workouts can help regulate sleep patterns and improve sleep quality, leading to more restful and rejuvenating sleep.

To reap the maximum benefits of cardio training, it's essential to choose activities that you enjoy and can sustain over time. Additionally, it's important to gradually increase the intensity and duration of your workouts to avoid overexertion and reduce the risk of injury. Incorporating a variety of cardio exercises into your fitness routine can help keep workouts engaging and prevent boredom.

Dr. Ian's Tip

PROTEIN SWAP

When protein consumption is mentioned, people automatically think of meat, particularly red meat. It's true that beef and chicken contain a tremendous amount of protein per serving, but there are other excellent sources of protein that are packaged with an array of health-promoting nutrients and are better for the environment. Legumes— the family of foods that includes beans, lentils, and peas— are nutritional powerhouses not only full of protein but also extremely affordable, versatile, and easy to find in most grocery stores. Load up on lentils, chickpeas, peas, soybeans, black beans, green beans, and get the protein you need along with a boost of energy.

COMPOUND EXERCISES

This type of exercise should be done during every decade. Compound exercises are called such because they involve more than one joint and use several muscle groups at once. For example, when you squat, you are bending at both the knees and hips and using several muscles, such as glutes, quads, hamstrings, calves, and core. These exercises are extremely efficient and will not only build muscle but save you workout time. The specific type of compound exercise you do can depend on many variables including age, fitness level, and ability to perform the movement. If you can't do all the exercises listed for your decade, don't worry. Incorporate as many as you can into your overall workout plan, a sample of which you will find at the end of this chapter. I've listed only a few compound exercises in the table below, but there are many more not on this list that you can try.

COMPOUND EXERCISES

WITH WEIGHTS	WITHOUT WEIGHTS
Bench Press (with bar or dumbbells)	Bulgarian Split Squat
Bent-Over Row	Burpees
Hip Thrust with Barbell	Lateral Lunge
Reverse Lunge with Overhead Press	Pull-Up
Deadlift	Push-Up
Bulgarian Split Squat with Dumbbells	Reverse Lunge with Knee Drive
Burpee Squat Press	Single-Leg Deadlift
Shoulder Press	Squat
Squat	Step-Up
Dumbbell Thrusters	Walking Lunge

Use this QR code to see videos of how these exercises are performed:

CORE EXERCISES

Core exercises are workouts that target the muscles in your abdomen, lower back, pelvis, and hips. Strengthening these muscles can improve stability, balance, posture, and overall athletic performance. Examples of core exercises include:

- **Plank:** Hold a push-up position, resting on your forearms and toes, keeping your body in a straight line.
- **Russian twist:** Sit on the floor with your knees bent, lean back slightly, and twist your torso from side to side, holding a weight or medicine ball.
- **Bicycle crunches:** Lie on your back, lift your legs, and perform a cycling motion while touching your opposite elbow to your knee.
- **Superman:** Lie face down on the floor, extend your arms and legs, then lift your arms, chest, and legs off the ground, engaging your lower back and glutes.
- **Mountain climber:** Begin in a push-up position, then alternate bringing each knee toward your chest in a running motion.
- **Dead bug:** Lie on your back with your arms extended toward the ceiling and legs raised, then lower opposite arm and leg toward the ground while keeping your back pressed against the floor.
- **Side plank:** Support your body on one forearm and the side of one foot, keeping your body in a straight line, and hold the position. Change sides.

Use this QR code to see how to perform these exercises:

HIGH-IMPACT EXERCISES

High-impact exercises are physical activities that put significant stress on your bones and joints due to the force of gravity. These exercises typically involve both feet leaving the ground simultaneously, causing a jolt to the body upon landing. While high-impact exercises can be great for cardiovascular health, bone density, and overall fitness, they may not be suitable for everyone, especially those with joint issues or injuries, so check with your doctor first. Some examples of high-impact exercises include jogging, running, jumping rope, tennis, racquetball, pickleball, mountain climbing, cardio kickboxing, aerobic dance classes, and plyometric exercises that involve explosive movements that rapidly stretch and contract muscles (box jumps, squat jumps, burpees, etc.).

HIGH-INTENSITY INTERVAL TRAINING (HIIT)

HIIT involves alternating between short bursts of high-intensity exercise and brief periods of rest or lower-intensity exercise. The idea is to push your body to its maximum effort during the high-intensity intervals, which can last anywhere from 20 seconds to several minutes, followed by a recovery period that allows your heart rate to come down before starting the next intense interval. During a HIIT session, you can choose from a variety of exercises, including cardiovascular exercises like running, cycling, jumping rope, or bodyweight exercises like burpees, mountain climbers, and high knees (running in place with knees thrusting high). The key is to perform each exercise at maximum effort during the high-intensity intervals and to allow yourself to recover during the rest periods.

The key benefits of HIIT include:

- **Increased calorie burn:** These workouts can help you burn more calories in a shorter amount of time compared to steady-state cardio exercises.

- **Improved cardiovascular health:** HIIT has been shown to improve cardiovascular health by increasing heart function and oxygen uptake.
- **Time efficiency:** These workouts are typically shorter than traditional cardio workouts because of the intensity level, making them ideal for people with busy schedules.
- **Increased metabolic rate:** HIIT can boost your metabolism, leading to continued calorie burn even after the workout is complete.
- **Adaptability:** These workouts can be tailored to individual fitness levels and preferences, making them accessible to people of all fitness levels.

LOW-IMPACT EXERCISES

Low-impact exercises refer to physical activities that place minimal stress on the joints, ligaments, and bones. These exercises are designed to be gentle on the body while still providing effective cardiovascular, strength, and flexibility benefits. These exercises typically involve controlled movements and moderate levels of intensity. Unlike high-impact exercises, which involve activities like running, jumping, or intense aerobics that can put significant strain on the joints and may increase the risk of injury, low-impact exercises are suitable for individuals of all fitness levels, including those with joint pain, arthritis, or other musculoskeletal conditions.

By choosing exercises that minimize joint impact, you can still engage in physical activity without exacerbating existing conditions or causing undue discomfort. Low-impact exercises can also be an excellent option for individuals recovering from injuries or surgeries, as they provide a safe and gradual way to rebuild strength and mobility. Overall, low-impact exercises offer a safe, effective, and enjoyable way to stay active and promote lifelong health and wellness.

Some examples include cycling, dancing, elliptical training, Pilates, rowing, swimming/water aerobics, Tai Chi, walking, and yoga.

PILATES

Pilates is a form of exercise that focuses on strengthening muscles while improving postural alignment and flexibility. It typically involves a series of precise movements performed on a mat or using specialized equipment, such as a reformer, Cadillacs, and barrels. Pilates is a holistic exercise system developed by Joseph Pilates in the early twentieth century. It emphasizes the integration of mind and body, with a focus on strengthening core muscles, improving flexibility, and enhancing overall body awareness and control.

One of the core principles of Pilates is breath control, where practitioners coordinate their movements with deep, rhythmic breathing patterns to promote relaxation, concentration, and efficient energy flow throughout the body. The exercises are designed to engage the deep stabilizing muscles of the abdomen, pelvis, and lower back, commonly referred to as the "powerhouse," which helps to improve posture, stability, and alignment.

Pilates exercises are often low impact, making them suitable for people of all fitness levels, ages, and body types. They can be adapted to meet individual needs and goals, whether it's rehabilitation from injury, enhancing athletic performance, or simply improving overall fitness and well-being.

POSTURAL TRAINING

Postural exercises are movements designed to improve posture by strengthening muscles, increasing flexibility, and promoting proper alignment of the body. They strengthen the core muscles, which, in turn, helps support proper posture. Some examples include:

- **Plank:** Get in a push-up position with your feet together and toes planted in the ground. Keep your arms straight and hands slightly wider than your shoulders. Your body from the middle of your shoulders down to your heels should be in a relatively straight line. A form variation is to rest your forearms on the ground rather than support yourself with your hands on the ground.
- **Wall angel:** Stand with your back against a wall and slowly raise your arms overhead while keeping your elbows and wrists in contact with the wall.
- **Cat-cow stretch:** Get on your hands and knees, arch your back up like a cat, then lower your belly and lift your head and tailbone like a cow.
- **Shoulder blade squeeze:** Sit or stand with arms at your sides, then squeeze your shoulder blades together while keeping your shoulders down.
- **Chin tuck:** Sit or stand tall, then gently tuck your chin toward your chest, lengthening the back of your neck.
- **Hip flexor stretch:** Kneel on one leg and slowly lunge forward, stretching the hip flexors of the back leg. Repeat on other leg.
- **Thoracic extension:** Lie down on the floor with a foam roller behind your midback. Clasp your hands behind your head. Slowly arch your back over the roller as you lower the back of your head toward the floor to stretch and mobilize the thoracic spine. Make sure to keep your feet and buttocks on the floor during the entire stretch.

Use this QR code to see how these exercises are performed:

STRENGTH TRAINING

Strength training, also known as resistance training, is a type of physical activity that uses resistance to improve muscle strength, endurance, and size. It typically involves lifting weights, using resistance bands, or using bodyweight exercises like push-ups and squats. The goal is to progressively overload the muscles, causing them to adapt and become stronger over time. Strength training can benefit overall health, increase metabolism, improve bone density, and enhance athletic performance.

There are many factors that go into how much weight you should be lifting as well as the number of repetitions and sets. All of us have unique requirements, goals, and abilities. It's best to consult a fitness expert/personal trainer to get guidance on what you should be lifting and how often, as well as what is safe for you. A general rule you might apply is to lift the amount of weight or resistance that challenges you and allows you to do enough repetitions, and stopping when you feel like you can only do 1 to 3 more repetitions. For example, if you're curling a 25-pound dumbbell and the most repetitions you can perform before losing proper form or unable to complete the full motion is 12, then you should only do 9 to 11 repetitions per set. Figuring out the ideal weight and repetitions for each exercise may take a little trial and error, but once you have established these numbers and feel comfortable, you will be able to gauge whether you're making progress.

If you have the means to work with a fitness expert or professional trainer for a few sessions, that can be extremely beneficial because you will learn how to train with proper form. Safety and efficacy are important when strength training, so don't just jump right into it; rather, get some guidance so that you can become knowledgeable about how to perform the exercises safely and effectively, and understand how to set realistic goals.

STRETCHING

Taking the time to stretch your body several times a week can be extremely beneficial. There are all kinds of quality stretching videos you can find online. The key, however, is consistency. Keeping your soft tissues loose and your extremities as limber as possible provides many important health benefits including:

- **Improved flexibility:** Increase your range of motion, which allows you to move more freely and perform daily activities with greater ease.
- **Reduced risk of injury:** Improve your muscle elasticity and joint mobility, which can reduce the likelihood of strains, sprains, and other injuries.
- **Enhanced athletic performance:** By increasing flexibility and range of motion, stretching can improve athletic performance and agility, leading to better overall sports performance.
- **Enhanced coordination and balance:** Stretching exercises that target stabilizing muscles can improve coordination and balance, reducing the risk of falls and enhancing overall stability.
- **Improved circulation:** Stretching increases blood flow to the muscles, which can help improve circulation and promote faster recovery after workouts.

- **Stress relief:** Stretching can help relax tense muscles and promote feelings of relaxation and well-being, making it an effective stress-relieving technique.
- **Better posture:** Stretching tight muscles can help correct imbalances in the body, leading to improved posture and reduced discomfort or pain.

YOGA

Yoga is a multifaceted discipline that originated in ancient India and has evolved over thousands of years. It encompasses physical, mental, and spiritual practices aimed at achieving harmony and balance within oneself and with the surrounding environment.

The physical aspect of yoga involves performing various postures or asanas, which are designed to stretch, strengthen, and align the body. These postures can range from gentle stretches to more challenging poses that require strength and flexibility. Through regular practice, yoga helps improve flexibility, mobility, and posture, reducing the risk of injuries and promoting overall physical health.

In addition to the physical postures, yoga incorporates breathing techniques known as pranayama. Pranayama techniques focus on controlling the breath to enhance vitality and promote relaxation. By learning to regulate the breath, practitioners can calm the mind, reduce stress, and improve concentration and focus.

Meditation is another integral component of yoga practice. Meditation involves training the mind to cultivate awareness, presence, and inner peace. Through meditation, practitioners learn to observe their thoughts without judgment, cultivate mindfulness, and develop a deeper understanding of themselves and their surroundings.

Yoga also emphasizes relaxation and stress reduction through practices such as deep relaxation (Savasana) and guided imagery. These practices help alleviate physical tension, calm the nervous system, and promote a sense of tranquility and well-being.

The benefits of yoga extend beyond the physical and mental realms to encompass spiritual growth and self-discovery. Many practitioners find that yoga provides a pathway for connecting with their inner selves, cultivating compassion and gratitude, and experiencing a deeper sense of purpose and fulfillment in life. It offers a comprehensive approach to health and wellness by addressing the interconnectedness of the body, mind, and spirit. Whether practiced for physical fitness, stress relief, spiritual growth, or all of the above, yoga provides a versatile and accessible tool for promoting holistic well-being.

4 MAJOR MOVEMENTS

There are four major movements that you will focus on—press, pull, knee flexion, and hinge. There are various exercises that can accomplish these four types of movement. It's important to incorporate a variety of exercises when trying to maximize improvements, so keep changing up your workouts. Make sure to choose the exercises that are safe for you based on your physical fitness level and capability.

Scan this QR code to see how these exercises are performed:

MOVEMENT	MUSCLES WORKED	EXERCISES
Press	Biceps Deltoids (anterior) Forearms Pectoralis Major Pectoralis Minor Serratus Anterior Trapezius Triceps	Bench Press Dumbbell Bench Press Dumbbell Lateral Raises Push-Ups Overhead Shoulder Press Chest Fly Chest Press (machine) Resistance Band Chest Press Triceps Dips Triceps Push-Downs
Pull	Back Biceps Forearms Deltoids (rear) Trapezius	Barbell Biceps Curls Barbell Shrugs Deadlifts Dumbbell Shrugs Hammer Curls Lat Pull-Downs Pull-Ups Rope Face Pulls Seated Cable Row Single-Arm TRX Row Single-Arm Dumbbell Bent-Over Row
Knee Flexion	Gastrocnemius Gracilis Hamstrings Plantaris Popliteus Sartorius	Bulgarian Split Squat Cycling Lunges (traditional and with barbells) Seated Knee Flexion Machine Squat (with/without weight) Standing Knee Flexion (with/without resistance) Wall Squat

Hip Hinge	Adductors
	Core
	Hamstrings
	Glutes
	Lower Back
	Quadriceps
	Upper Back
		Barbell Hip Thrust
		Bodyweight Hip Thrust
		Cable Pull-Throughs
		Deadlift with
		  Barbell/Kettlebell/Dumbbells
		Glute Bridge
		Goblet Squat
		Kettlebell Swing
		Single-Leg Deadlift
		  (with/without Kettlebell)

YOUR PLAN

Everyone has a different level of experience, ability, strength, and endurance. Goals can also be very different based on many variables. Thus, no one plan is perfect for everyone. This plan is a general concept of how you might structure your workout to incorporate as many of the exercises as possible that will help you achieve results in many areas, including strength, endurance, mobility, flexibility, performance, and range of motion. This is just a beginning plan. You can modify it according to your goals, needs, and progress. You can add more sets as you get stronger and better conditioned. You can increase the weight by 10 percent if you're using resistance for some of the exercises. Make sure you choose different exercises to do for the different sessions. There are all kinds of customizations you can make to the plan that will suit your needs. The most important thing is to use the plan as a guideline and make it work for you. The purpose of this plan is to simply give you a broad idea of how you can assemble a workout strategy that can work for your abilities and goals.

30S

Do 2 press workouts each week:
- Choose 3 exercises from the press category for each workout.
- Do 3 sets of each exercise per workout.
- **Example workout session:** 3 sets of bench presses, 3 sets of chest flys, 3 sets of triceps push-downs

Do 2 pull workouts each week:
- Choose 3 exercises from the pull category for each workout.
- Do 3 sets of each exercise per workout.

- **Example workout session:** 3 sets of biceps curls, 3 sets of pull-ups, 3 sets of seated cable rows

Do at least 1 knee flexion workout each week:
- Choose 3 exercises from the knee flexion category for each workout.
- Do 3 sets of each exercise per workout.
- **Example workout session:** 3 sets of squats, 3 sets of seated leg flex machine, 3 sets of lunges

Do 2 hip hinge workouts each week:
- Choose 3 exercises from the hip hinge category for each workout.
- Do 3 sets of each exercise per workout.
- **Example workout session:** 3 sets of glute bridges, 3 sets of goblet squats, 3 sets of kettle bell swings

Do two 20- to 30-minute cardio sessions each week:
- Feel free to break this up into smaller sessions, such as 15 minutes in the morning and 15 minutes in the afternoon/evening

40S

Do 1 press workout each week:
- Choose 3 exercises from the press category for each workout.
- Do 3 sets of each exercise per workout.
- **Example workout session:** 3 sets of bench presses, 3 sets of chest flys, 3 sets of triceps push-downs

Do 1 pull workout each week:
- Choose 3 exercises from the pull category for each workout.

- Do 3 sets of each exercise per workout.
- **Example workout session:** 3 sets of biceps curls, 3 sets of pull-ups, 3 sets of seated cable rows

Do at least 1 knee flexion workout each week:
- Choose 3 exercises from the knee flexion category for each workout.
- Do 3 sets of each exercise per workout.
- **Example workout session:** 3 sets of squats, 3 sets of seated leg flex machine, 3 sets of lunges

Do 1 hip hinge workout each week:
- Choose 3 exercises from the hip hinge category for each workout.
- Do 3 sets of each exercise per workout.
- **Example workout session:** 3 sets of glute bridges, 3 sets of goblet squats, 3 sets of kettle bell swings

Do two 20- to 30-minute cardio sessions each week:
- Feel free to break this up into smaller sessions, such as 15 minutes in the morning and 15 minutes in the afternoon/evening.
- You can also play a sport to fulfill these cardio sessions (racquetball, tennis, basketball, cycling, rowing, etc.).

50S

Do 1 press workout each week:
- Choose 3 exercises from the press category for each workout.
- Do 3 sets of each exercise per workout.
- **Example workout session:** 3 sets of bench presses, 3 sets of chest flys, 3 sets of triceps push-downs

Do 2 pull workouts each week:

- Choose 3 exercises from the pull category for each workout.
- Do 3 sets of each exercise per workout.
- **Example workout session:** 3 sets of biceps curls, 3 sets of pull-ups, 3 sets of seated cable rows

Do at least 1 knee flexion workout each week:

- Choose 3 exercises from the knee flexion category for each workout.
- Do 3 sets of each exercise per workout.
- **Example workout session:** 3 sets of squats, 3 sets of seated leg flex machine, 3 sets of lunges

Do 2 hip hinge workouts each week:

- Choose 3 exercises from the hip hinge category for each workout.
- Do 3 sets of each exercise per workout.
- **Example workout session:** 3 sets of glute bridges, 3 sets of goblet squats, 3 sets of kettle bell swings

Do two 20- to 30-minute cardio sessions each week:

- Feel free to break this up into smaller sessions, such as 15 minutes in the morning and 15 minutes in the afternoon/evening.

60s+

Do 1 press workout each week:

- Choose 3 exercises from the press category for each workout.
- Do 3 sets of each exercise per workout.
- **Example workout session:** 3 sets of bench presses, 3 sets of chest flys, 3 sets of triceps push-downs

Do 1 pull workout each week:
- Choose 3 exercises from the pull category for each workout.
- Do 3 sets of each exercise per workout.
- **Example workout session:** 3 sets of biceps curls, 3 sets of pull-ups, 3 sets of seated cable rows

Do at least 1 knee flexion workout each week:
- Choose 3 exercises from the knee flexion category for each workout.
- Do 3 sets of each exercise per workout.
- **Example workout session:** 3 sets of squats, 3 sets of seated leg flex machine, 3 sets of lunges

Do 1 hip hinge workout each week:
- Choose 3 exercises from the hip hinge category for each workout.
- Do 3 sets of each exercise per workout.
- **Example workout session:** 3 sets of glute bridges, 3 sets of goblet squats, 3 sets of kettle bell swings

Do two 20- to 30-minute cardio sessions each week:
- Feel free to break this up into smaller sessions, such as 15 minutes in the morning and 15 minutes in the afternoon/evening.

Do 2 postural sessions each week.

The Inspiration

Beverly is a 51-year-old accountant who is in generally good health but leads a largely sedentary lifestyle and has occasional joint pain. Beverly is not a big fan of the gym, and while she keeps promising herself that she is going to go back, she simply can't find the motivation to do so. Despite a lack of enthusiasm for traditional gym workouts, Beverly recognizes the importance of staying active for her overall health and well-being.

The Plan

Concerned about her fitness level, Beverly confided in her friend Hailey about her desire to find a more enjoyable form of exercise. Hailey suggested pickleball, a sport she recently started playing and finds both fun and effective for fitness. Intrigued by the idea, Beverly decided to give pickleball a try, seeing it as an opportunity to incorporate physical activity into her routine in a way that feels less like a chore.

Beverly joined Hailey for a few introductory pickleball sessions at a local community center. Initially, Beverly struggled with the basics of the game, but she enjoyed the social aspect and the opportunity to spend time outdoors. Despite the initial challenges, Beverly was determined to improve her skills and committed to practicing regularly.

The Change

Over the course of a few weeks, Beverly noticed significant improvements in her fitness levels and overall well-being. She experienced increased energy levels, improved mood, and reduced joint pain as she became more accustomed to the physical demands of pickleball. Beverly also began making healthier lifestyle choices, such as opting for nutritious meals and prioritizing sleep to support her active lifestyle. Her dedication to pickleball paid off as she not only improved her fitness levels but also discovered a newfound passion for the sport. Encouraged by her progress, Beverly set new goals for herself, aiming to participate in local pickleball tournaments and further refine her skills. The sense of achievement and camaraderie she experiences through pickleball serve as powerful motivators for Beverly to continue prioritizing her health and fitness. Her journey highlights the importance of finding enjoyable forms of exercise to maintain long-term adherence to physical activity goals. By embracing pickleball as her preferred method of staying active, Beverly not only achieved her initial goal of improving fitness but also discovered a fulfilling and sustainable way to incorporate exercise into her lifestyle. Through dedication and perseverance, Beverly proved that age is no barrier to pursuing new passions and prioritizing health and well-being.

8

THE BODY FIX

An inevitable part of aging is the change in not only how our body looks but also in how it works. Our body is composed of billions of cells, over 600 muscles, 206 bones, and 78 organs. While the body might be the most ingenious machine ever constructed, it still is vulnerable to the wear and tear consequences of repeated use. Some parts can be rejuvenated and replaced with newer versions, but many cannot. This means that as we age, we naturally increase the exhaustion of our cells, organs, and tissues.

The signs of aging are well documented—you may notice sagging, wrinkled skin, gray and thinning hair, curvature of the spine, hunched shoulders, hollow cheeks, reduced muscle mass, and a slower and less steady gait. While it's certainly no fun to experience these changes, many of these age-related characteristics can be slowed or prevented by making smart choices. You might not be able to totally avoid wrinkles and sagging areas of skin, but you can definitely delay their onset and quantity. It's unlikely you will be able to run a mile as quickly in your late 60s as you did in your early 30s, but that doesn't mean you have to be relegated to only walking as you age. In this chapter, you will find some of the most common body changes for each decade of life and ways you might be able to fix them. However, don't just focus on your decade; rather, look at the others to see what's possibly in your future and adopt small changes in your daily life now that will help you prevent or combat the severity of what's to come.

30S	40S	50S	60S+
Decreased Bone Density	Decreased Bone Density	Decreased Bone Density	Decreased Bone Density
Cardiovascular Fitness Decline	Cardiovascular Fitness Decline	Heart Muscle Weakens	Decreased Brain Size
Decreased Flexibility	Buttocks Muscle Atrophy	Thinning Joints	Decreased Flexibility
Muscle Mass Loss	Decreased Flexibility	Muscle Loss	Heart Dysfunction
Weight Gain	Muscle Mass Loss	Perimenopause/ Menopause	Joint Deterioration
	Perimenopause/ Menopause	Changing Skin (dryness, sagging, uneven skin tone, thinning, spotting)	Diminished Lung Capacity
	Skin Changes (thinning, wrinkling, sagging, spotting)	Weight Gain	Muscle Mass Loss
	Vision Impairment		Skin Changes (age spots, bruising, deep wrinkling
	Weight Gain		

Dr. Ian's Tips

SNACK SMART

Snacks between meals are great opportunities for a healthy energy boost, but they're often wasted. Sure, a couple of chocolate chip cookies or a slice of pie are always mouth-watering, but they should be balanced with snacks such as vegetables and hummus, yogurt and granola, cheese and tomatoes—snack choices that not only taste great but can give you a boost of energy, a feeling of fullness, and nutrients to improve your health. If you plan to have three snacks over the course of the day, make a deal with yourself. Allow one of those snacks to be your favorite treat, and commit to making the other two snacks beneficial: to quash those hunger pangs but also provide a quick injection of healthiness.

THE 30s

There are few major changes your body will go through in your 30s as a result of the aging process, but those that do occur should be monitored closely. If these early physical and functional changes are ignored or not addressed proactively, they could become bigger problems for you in the future. When it comes to your health, remember that it's much better to stay ahead of the game than try to play catch-up.

Body Changes

Decreased bone density   Muscle loss
Cardiovascular decline   Weight gain
Decreased flexibility

DECREASED BONE DENSITY

According to the American Academy of Orthopaedic Surgeons, most people will reach their peak bone mass somewhere between the ages of 25 and 30. Once this peak is reached, bone mass stays consistent for some time, then around age 40, it slowly starts to diminish. For some, this bone density loss might happen sooner or slightly later. For everyone, however, as we age, the rate of bone thinning will increase if nothing is done to stop it or slow it down. At the microscopic level, our bones are in a constant state of being created and destroyed. Bone is laid down and bone is resorbed. As we grow older, however, the laying down process doesn't keep up with the resorption process, so the bones become progressively thinner. If you add other risk factors, such as smoking, inadequate calcium or vitamin D intake, lack of weight-bearing exercise, and a disrupted hormonal environment (low estrogen in women and low testosterone in men), bone density decline is accelerated.

Fix It

At this stage of life, it's important to get ahead before you fall behind. The two most important things you can do to keep your bones healthy are exercise and consuming enough calcium. Choose weight-bearing exercises that have an impact on the body's physical skeleton, such as brisk walking, jogging or running, stair climbing, dancing, and using weight machines, resistance bands, body weight workouts (push-ups, pull-ups, jumping jacks), and free weights. Make sure you're getting enough calcium, that all-important mineral that keeps your bones strong. Both men and women should consume at least 1,000 mg of calcium each day. Vitamin D is also critical as it helps the body absorb the calcium and phosphorus that is stored in our bones and makes them stronger and more durable. If you are a smoker, stop. If you are not a smoker, don't start. Smoking can increase your risk for weakening bones. Lastly, limit your alcohol consumption—if you drink at all, drink only in moderation. Excessive alcohol consumption can cause harm to many of your organs, including the liver, brain, and bones.

CARDIOVASCULAR DECLINE

This is the decade when you might first notice a decline in your physical stamina. You might start getting winded from physical activities (climbing stairs, running after small children, carrying heavy boxes) that didn't challenge you in the past. Your heart and lungs need to work together during physical activity, and when they have not been adequately challenged through exercise or physical activity, they get out of synch and the result is you find it difficult to breathe comfortably during moments of increased exertion. Remember, your heart is a muscle, and it must be exercised just like other muscles in your body to maintain its strength and level of functioning.

Fix It

Consume foods that are lower in fat and calories and higher in antioxidants and whole grains. Keep your cholesterol levels in check to prevent the buildup of plaque (atherosclerosis) on the inside of your blood vessels. Maintain or improve your aerobic fitness by doing high-intensity interval training (HIIT) three times a week. This will exercise your heart, causing it to beat faster for short periods of time, then giving it time to slow down before prompting it to beat faster again when you increase your exertion.

DECREASED FLEXIBILITY

There are many reasons why your body starts to lose its flexibility during this decade. If you have a job that requires sitting all day, your muscles and other soft tissues likely aren't being stretched enough to maintain their ability to lengthen on demand. The physical activities you might be doing, such as weightlifting, running, or playing soccer, don't regularly put your body through a full range of motion at the various joints in your body. Soft tissues must be stretched, and joints must be fully opened on a regular basis to keep your body limber and supple.

Fix It

Foam rollers, which might look very simple and unsophisticated, can be extremely helpful in stretching out those cranky soft tissues. They are cylindrical pieces of foam over which a body part is rolled to help release the tension in soft tissues. Muscles are covered by fascia, a thin layer of connective tissue that also embeds itself throughout the muscle fibers. Both the muscles and the fascia can tighten as you age or if you are injured. Besides using a foam roller, there are other techniques and devices that can help you achieve myofascial release and regain flexibility. Roll the targeted areas up and down over the foam roller several times a week for just a few minutes.

MUSCLE LOSS

The beauty and advantage of youth is that during these years, the body has the amazing ability to heal, repair, grow, and flourish despite how badly it's treated or neglected. There's a physical resiliency and forgiveness that exists when we're young that doesn't exist in our older years. Our muscle volume and strength can become victims of age if they are not exercised and nourished properly, and your 30s is typically the first decade of life when most people start noticing it. Many are well into establishing their careers, and their lives are busy with familial and social obligations. Time is at a premium, and exercise often slides down the priority list. Muscles are very needy tissues. They need nourishment, activity, and attention to maintain or grow their strength and size. "Use it or lose it"—this adage perfectly describes the fate of your muscles, and this is the decade to really start using them.

Fix It

Adopt an exercise regimen that includes resistance training at least three times a week. This training can incorporate resistance bands, free weights, weight machines, or body-weight exercises. You don't need to spend hours exercising your muscles. Focused, 30-minute sessions with the proper lifting technique and workout strategy can be enough to give your muscles the necessary stimulation they need to maintain their size or grow. Muscles are also made in the kitchen, so make sure you are eating plenty of lean protein—animal and/or plant—because protein is the building block of healthy muscle.

WEIGHT GAIN

People gain weight at different rates and at different times in their life. Researchers looked at data from more than 13,000 people in the National Health and Nutrition Examination Survey and published their findings in the *Journal of Obesity*.[1] They wanted to determine at what age people put on the most pounds. The study found that, on average, adults gained 17.6 pounds from their late 20s to the late 30s and 14.3 pounds during their 30s and 40s. On average, women gained more weight than men during a 10-year period, putting on an average of 12 pounds compared with 6 pounds for men. Researchers found that the most weight gain occurs in young and middle-aged adults, and the older we get, the less weight is gained. While weight gain in your 30s might not tip the scale into obesity, it can put you on an undesirable path. This is the time to be determined and proactive to avoid potential myriad weight-related health problems that will not only impact how you live but can also be expensive when considering the cost of treatment and potential loss of work opportunities due to illness and health-related restrictions. In this decade, work, family life, social obligations, and financial concerns become priorities, which could lead to a more sedentary lifestyle with less time for physical activities. When physical activity diminishes and calorie consumption stays the same or increases, weight gain is inevitable. Now is the time to do something as it becomes more difficult to address weight gain as we age.

Fix It

Build a successful weight management program that involves both a specific nutrition plan as well as an exercise regimen. There are many weight-loss strategies that have proven effective, but the most important thing is that you choose a plan that works for you. Make sure the food on the plan is affordable, accessible, and meets your taste preferences, and the eating strategy (low carbs, intermittent fasting, modified keto) is one that you can do consistently for a long period of time. Your exercise regimen should have certain elements. You should exercise a minimum of three times a week. Your workouts should include both strength training and cardiovascular exercises. At a minimum, do two cardio sessions of 20 to 30 minutes in duration and two strength training sessions. One of these cardio sessions should be high-intensity interval training (HIIT). Look at chapter 7 to see some of your top exercises. It's less about how much time you're in the gym and more about the quality of time you spend while exercising. You can get a good-quality workout in just 20 minutes if you're doing the right exercises in the right way. Use the QR code below to connect to my fitness app that will provide you with over a hundred instructional videos that will help get your fitness game on point.

THE 40s

It's likely that most people will hit their 40s without experiencing any major medical problems. Sure, there could be a broken bone from a sports injury or an infection that needs antibiotics, even a diagnosis of prediabetes. However, issues such as heart attacks, strokes, or major neurological dysfunction are not likely to happen. This decade, however, can be one of those important inflection points for one's health journey. Years of unhealthy habits, neglected self-care, chaotic schedules, and poor lifestyle choices can start taking their toll. We start noticing aches and pains that don't seem to go away as quickly as they used to. Healing from injuries takes longer. Our reflexes tend to be a tad slower. Energy levels start to dip, and activities that we were once able to participate in without any difficulty may become somewhat more challenging. The time when we could consistently eat 1,500-calorie meals and not suffer any repercussions has passed, and these calorie-rich meals can start to show up on our waistline and the number on the scale may be increasing. Women start entering perimenopause and experiencing all the physiological changes that come with it. Some of these changes involve a drop in estrogen levels, which can have several consequences, including irregular menstruation, a loss of sexual drive and difficulty getting aroused, and hot flashes. Men may start to notice the effects of lower testosterone levels with their libido dipping and their sexual performance not as vigorous as it has been in the past. Muscle mass tends to decline while the number on the scale starts sneaking upward. This is a decade of change and a time when many people need to make wholesale changes to get back on a healthy course or find themselves on an unfortunate trajectory of physical deterioration and its related health consequences.

Body Changes

Decreased bone density	Decreased flexibility
Butt sags	Muscle loss

Perimenopause/
  menopause
Skin changes (thinning,
  wrinkling, sagging,
  spotting)

Vision impairment
Weight gain

DECREASED BONE DENSITY

Once bone mass has peaked in your early 30s, there's a period in which it stays consistent, then starts to decline. This is a decade where, if nothing is done to slow the rate of bone loss, our bones start losing their mineralization at the microscopic level. Eventually, as we continue to age, they become thinner and more prone to fractures. Lifestyle behaviors (smoking, poor calcium and vitamin D intake, lack of weight-bearing exercises) can accelerate the bone loss, so this is a decade where it's important to maintain good bone stock rather than contribute to weakening it.

Fix It

Similar to what is helpful in your 30s, it's important to get ahead before you fall behind. Exercise and adequate calcium consumption are two of the most important things that can create an environment for healthy bones. Your bones are primed to remain healthy when they are physically challenged through weight-bearing exercises, such as brisk walking, jogging or running, stair climbing, dancing, using weight machines, resistance bands, and free weights, and doing bodyweight workouts (push-ups, pull-ups, jumping jacks). Make sure you're getting enough calcium, that all-important mineral that keeps your bones strong. Both men and women should consume at least 1,000 mg of calcium each day. Vitamin D is also critical as it helps the body absorb the calcium and phosphorus that are stored in our bones and makes them stronger and more durable. Avoid smoking and limit your alcohol consumption as both can contribute to weaker bones. It's important to remember that beyond impacting your bone health, excessive alcohol consumption can harm organs, such as your liver and brain.

BUTT SAGS

A large determiner of the size and shape of our butt is our genetics. However, how these genes manifest is partially in our control. The major contributors to the shape of our buttocks are the gluteal muscles (glutes) and fat, with muscles playing the most important part. As we age, if our glutes aren't being activated properly and frequently enough, the muscles start to atrophy, and the shape starts to transform from one that is more rounded and fuller to one that is flatter and more concave. There are three gluteal muscles—gluteus maximus, gluteus medius, and gluteus minimus. The gluteus maximus is the largest of the three and comprises most of the shape and form of the butt. Fat is also a player in the desirable plumpness, but just like muscle, it atrophies (thins and shrinks) as we age. This, combined with skin losing elasticity as we age, also contributes to the flattening and sagging of the derriere. The good news is that there are things you can do to prevent or decrease the amount of flattening that occurs as we age, and it has nothing to do with undergoing a plastic surgeon's knife.

Fix It

Maintaining or improving the shape of your butt comes down to one thing: exercise! Here are five exercises you can do for just three 15-minute sessions per week that will help prevent sagging or return that lifted shape you desire.

1. **Donkey kicks.** Start on the ground on your hands and knees with your hands placed directly under your shoulders. Bend one leg up behind you while the other knee stays on the ground. Make sure the foot of the leg that is raised remains parallel to the ground. Raise your leg up so that your knee is parallel to your butt, making sure you really squeeze your glutes at the top of the motion. Bring your leg back down with your knee coming almost even with the other one that has remained on the ground, then go back up again. Make sure you keep your back flat throughout the entire motion and breathe evenly. Do this for 10 repetitions on one side, then do the same on the other leg. Do four sets of 10 repetitions with each leg.

2. **Squats.** Grab a pair of dumbbells in each hand. Choose a weight that you can comfortably hold for the completion of the exercise (10 repetitions) without losing your form. Spread your legs a little wider than your shoulders with your toes facing directly forward or slightly angled outward. Bend your knees and squat down as if sitting in a chair. Once your knees reach 90 degrees (right angle) then come back up, squeezing your glutes as you finish standing erectly. Complete four sets of 10 squats.

3. **Glute bridge.** Lie flat on your back with knees bent and feet flat. Transfer all your weight into your heels, using them as your thrust points. Press your heels into the ground and at the same time lift your hips so that they are at equal height with your knees. Do this for 10 repetitions. Do four sets.

4. **Fire hydrant.** This is named after the motion dogs make when peeing on a fire hydrant. Keep that visual of them standing next to it and lifting one leg up to the side as they do their business. Take a lightweight resistance band and wrap it around your legs just above your knees. Get on your knees as if you were doing donkey kicks. The difference between this and the donkey kick is that instead

of lifting your leg up behind you, lift your leg up to the side (like a dog peeing on a fire hydrant) as high as you can. Keep your back straight and your trunk as quiet as possible so that the work is concentrated on the upper and outer portion of your butt. Squeeze your glutes at the top of the motion. Compete 10 repetitions for each set and do four sets.

5. **Split squat.** Take a large step forward with your left foot, making sure your weight is evenly distributed over both feet. Place both hands on the sides of your hips. Bend your knees as you squat down toward the ground, stopping when your right knee is a few inches above the ground. Stand back up to the starting position, then repeat the squat. Do 10 repetitions, then switch leg positions and do 10 repetitions with the other leg forward. Do four sets with each leg forward.

Use this QR code to see videos of these exercises:

DECREASED FLEXIBILITY

Our muscles and soft tissues need to be able to relax and stretch at various times; however, as we age, these tissues become less flexible, which can result in stress on other body parts. When muscles are tight and don't stretch and relax properly, our range of motion becomes limited. Like in your 30s, there are many reasons why your body starts to lose its flexibility during this decade. If you have an office job or one that requires sitting all day, your muscles and other soft tissues aren't being stretched like they need to be to maintain their ability to lengthen on demand. The physical activities you might be doing don't regularly put your body through a full range of motion at the various joints in your body, which means your muscles and joints aren't being challenged frequently enough. Soft tissues must be stretched, and joints must be fully opened on a regular basis to keep your body limber and supple.

Fix It

Here are three simple types of exercise that can maintain and improve your flexibility.

1. **Dynamic stretching.** These are stretches that gently move joints through their full range of motion in a controlled manner. They increase blood flow to the muscles and other soft tissues, increasing muscle temperature and decreasing muscle stiffness. These are great stretches to do as part of a warm-up routine before any athletic or sporting event. Some examples of these stretches are arm helicopters, leg swings, walking lunges, torso twists, walking hip rotators.

2. **Foam rolling.** While foam rollers may look simple and unsophisticated, they can be extremely helpful in stretching out those cranky soft tissues. Muscles are covered by fascia, a thin layer of connective tissue that also embeds itself throughout the muscle fibers. Both the muscles and the fascia can tighten as you age or if you are injured. Besides using a foam roller, there are other techniques and devices that can help you achieve myofascial release and regain flexibility. Roll the targeted areas up and down over the foam roller several times a week for just a few minutes.

3. **Static stretches.** Unlike dynamic stretching, where you actively move your joints through a full range of motion,

these stretches involve standing, sitting, or lying still while holding a single stretched position for 30 seconds or more. Once you have held the stretch for the desired time, release the position and remain in the relaxed state for a few seconds, then assume the stretched position again and hold for the desired time. Repeat this several times, then move to the next body part to be stretched. There are many examples of static stretching. Some of the more common ones include stretches of the hamstrings, hip flexors, calf, shoulders, neck, chest, triceps, wrist, spine, and quads.

Use this QR code to see videos of these stretches:

MUSCLE LOSS

Muscle mass is for more than just show and bragging rights on the beach. It is critical to how we move, how we function, and for our overall health. It's much easier to build muscle in our younger years simply because we tend to have higher protein levels and our physical activity levels tend to be higher and more suitable to what's needed to grow muscle. However, as we get older, our dietary and physical activity habits change, and these changes do not favor muscle maintenance or growth. In fact, it becomes even more critical that as we age we become more intentional about our protein intake. Experts suggest that we need even more protein than when we're young to help maintain our muscle mass; however, we tend to start eating less and becoming more sedentary, a combination that increases the risk of deteriorating muscle mass.

Fix It

Reversing muscle loss that's a result of aging and decreased physical activity is much easier than you might think. It doesn't require a lot of time, rather just a reasonable strategy, dedication, and consistency. Make sure to consult your doctor first, but here are some ways to maintain or improve your muscle mass during this decade.

1. **Resistance training.** Whether it's using free weights or resistance bands, establish a consistent strength training routine and do it two to three times per week for at least 30 minutes each session.

2. **Consume protein.** Protein contains amino acids, which are the building blocks of muscle. You need sufficient amounts of protein for your muscles to grow. There are plenty of healthy animal and nonanimal sources of protein (fish, chicken, beef, beans, legumes, yogurt, chia seeds) you can add to your daily diet that will help create a better muscle-building environment. Try to consume protein-rich foods within an hour after your workout to help with muscle repair and growth.

3. **Vitamin D.** Vitamin D is not only important in helping the body absorb and retain calcium and phosphorus to build strong bone, but it's also involved in the synthesis of protein, as well as increasing the size of muscle cells and muscle mass. Make sure your vitamin D levels are adequate, something that can be assessed through a simple blood test administered by your healthcare provider. If your levels are low, add more vitamin D–containing foods or consider taking supplements.

4. **Increase omega-3s.** Omega-3 fatty acids can do more than improve brain function and protect your heart. Studies have suggested that they can contribute to muscle growth because of their anti-inflammatory properties. It's believed that omega-3s play a role in muscle protein synthesis, reducing post-workout muscle soreness, improving workout quality, and slowing muscle loss due to aging. Omega-3s can be found in many foods, including fish such as mackerel and salmon, flaxseed, chia seeds, soybeans, and nuts. You can also get quality omega-3 supplements in a capsule or liquid form.

5. **Get more sleep.** One of the most important parts of muscle building is recovery. Proper nutrition is a critical part of recovery, but so is getting the appropriate amount of sleep. When we sleep, our body releases human growth hormone, which can help muscles grow and keep the stress hormone cortisol in check. Inadequate sleep can also lead to a decrease in muscle-building testosterone. How much sleep do you need? There is no one answer for everyone, but most sleep experts recommend at least 7 to 9 hours of sleep per night.

PERIMENOPAUSE/MENOPAUSE

Perimenopause is the time when a woman begins to transition into menopause. This transition typically begins between the ages of 45 and 55 and usually lasts about 7 years, but for some women it can go as long as 14 years. During perimenopause, the ovaries are still making estrogen but are gradually making less. When the ovaries stop releasing estrogen and the menstrual cycles stop, a woman is in full menopause. Many women start experiencing symptoms (hot flashes, racing heart, sweating, vaginal dryness, sore breasts, difficulty sleeping, emotional changes, dry skin) during perimenopause that might increase in frequency and intensity during menopause. Menopause is a biological inevitability, and it comes at different times and in different ways for all women. Being aware of your body and your symptoms can inform the steps you can take to make this a less challenging time in your life.

Fix It

You can't stop or avoid perimenopause or menopause, however, you can treat or limit the severity of some of the symptoms you experience. It's important to remember that many of these symptoms will go away over time, but if they are causing problems, there's no reason you can't try to mitigate their impact now. There are a number of treatments available, including hormone replacement therapy (HRT) and nonhormone medications such as paroxetine, gabapentin, clonidine, and selective estrogen receptor modulators (SERMS) that manage how estrogen works in the body by providing relief from hot flashes. Not all treatments work the same for everyone, and they should be taken under the supervision of or in consultation with your physician. There are many herbal supplements available, such as soy, maca, valerian root, red clover, and black cohosh, that have been promoted and reported as potentially being beneficial for certain symptoms. While most of the studies' results are mixed, many women describe anecdotally their positive experiences in using these supplements. Read about these treatments carefully, and make sure you get the advice of a healthcare professional before starting them.

SKIN CHANGES

Our skin is one of the first places where we start to see the effects of aging. These age-related skin changes, while not necessarily desirable, are still considered to be healthy changes because they are part of the normal process of getting older. Thinning, wrinkling, and sagging will happen to everyone who lives long enough to experience them. You will encounter areas of broken blood vessels, age spots, and dry patches. The most critical unhealthy skin change that can be experienced is skin cancer, which is why limiting exposure to the sun from an early age and wearing adequate sunscreen are essential starting in childhood. Skin cancer caused by excessive sun exposure is not a condition that develops overnight. Rather, years of poor skin protection can cause microdamage to the skin cells, and this damage accumulates and multiplies in its danger until the changes become cancerous. Regular skin self-checks are important. You can read more about these self-exams in chapter 9. There is plenty you can do to protect your skin and keep it looking younger without resorting to plastic surgery or invasive dermatological procedures. Some of these procedures might help in some cases, but they can also be expensive, and if done too often or by an unaccredited practitioner, they can create even more damage. Try some of the natural fixes below to keep your skin healthy.

Fix It

Here are some simple things you can do right away at home to help prevent or improve skin problems.

1. **Limit sun exposure/use sunscreen.** Avoid intense sun exposure for prolonged periods of time. Wear protective clothing and eyewear, making sure you cover the less obvious areas like the back of the neck, eyes, ears, and back of the arms and legs. Use a broad-spectrum sunscreen of at least SPF 30 and apply it generously over all areas that will be exposed to the sun. Typically, enough sunscreen to fill a shot glass should be sufficient; however, if you need to cover more of your body surface area, you might need to

use more sunscreen. Reapply every 2 hours or even more frequently if you are swimming or sweating.

2. **Moisturize regularly.** Applying moisturizer when the skin is slightly wet helps trap the water to be absorbed by the skin. Your skin can get dry in various climate conditions, so don't be afraid to moisturize twice a day if necessary.

3. **Use gentle skin products.** Make sure you use products that are pH-neutral, which means they are adapted to the pH of the skin. Our skin is slightly acidic, so products should match this. Avoid using perfumed soaps and taking long, hot showers, which can dry out your skin. Bathe in warm water, making sure to use mild cleansers that won't irritate your skin. Wash gently and be careful not to scrub your skin too hard. If you are using an exfoliant, make sure it's not so harsh that it leaves your skin raw and removes more than just the dry outer skin cells.

4. **Avoid sunlamps and tanning beds.** These machines can be extremely harmful to your skin. While you might like the appearance of being tan, tanning beds emit the same harmful UV radiation as the sun and can do as much damage if not more, depending on the machine's strength and amount of time you're exposed to it. Sunlamps have been used to treat many conditions, such as seasonal affective disorder (SAD), vitamin D deficiency, and mood swings. However, they should be used only after consulting with your doctor to determine what's safe for you.

5. **Avoid tobacco smoke.** Smoking tobacco and being exposed to it in high quantities can accelerate aging and damage your skin. Besides the dramatic cancer risk it poses, smoking changes not just the skin, but your teeth and hair in ways that make you look much older. Smoking causes the skin to be chronically deprived of oxygen and nutrients, thus making the skin appear pale, loose, and wrinkled, especially around the mouth and eyes.

VISION IMPAIRMENT

This is the decade when most adults will start noticing changes in their vision. Most commonly, seeing clearly at close distances becomes a challenge, especially when reading or looking at a device's screen. This condition, called presbyopia, is when the eyes gradually lose the ability to focus on nearby objects. Presbyopia will continue to slowly progress over time up until your mid-60s. You might experience other vision problems, such as difficulty seeing well in low light, reduced tear production, problems with glare from approaching headlights, and changes in color perception. Other eye problems that can arise during this decade, and that are potentially more dangerous, include macular degeneration and retina problems and are related to other health conditions, such as diabetes, high cholesterol, and thyroid abnormalities.

Fix It

Remedies for vision problems generally depend on the causes. You should have a full eye examination as a matter of course, even before you start noticing changes. Once the eye specialist has a diagnosis and a better grasp of what's going on, a treatment plan that could be as simple as acquiring reading glasses or a new prescription can be implemented. Some conditions that can have an impact on your vision, such as diabetes and hyperthyroidism, might require medication or other treatments such as surgery. Those suffering eye strain from looking at a computer or phone screen too long will need to change their viewing habits. All of these options can be discussed and worked out with your healthcare provider.

WEIGHT GAIN

People gain weight at different rates and at different times in their life. Researchers looked at data from more than 13,000 people in the National Health and Nutrition Examination Survey and published their findings in the *Journal of Obesity*.[2] They wanted to determine during which decades of life people put on the most pounds. The study found that, on average, adults gained approximately 14 pounds during their 40s. Women gained more than men—17 pounds for women compared to 11 pounds for men. Researchers found that for each successive decade, the weight gain decreased. The 30s, 40s, and 50s decades showed the most weight gain and in that order. While your weight gain during this decade might not tip the scale into obesity, it might put you on an undesirable path. This is the time to be determined and proactive to avoid potential myriad weight-related health problems that will not only impact how you live but can also be expensive when considering the cost of treatment and potential loss of work opportunities due to illness and health-related restrictions.

Fix It

Build a successful weight management program that involves both a specific nutrition plan as well as an exercise regimen. There are many weight-loss strategies that have proven effective, but the most important thing is that you wisely choose a plan that will work for you. Make sure the food on the plan is affordable, accessible, and meets your taste preferences, and that the eating strategy (low carbs, intermittent fasting, modified keto) is one that you can do consistently for a long period of time. Your exercise regimen should have certain elements. You should exercise a minimum of three times a week. Your workouts should include both strength training and cardiovascular exercises. At a minimum, do two cardio sessions of 20 to 30 minutes in duration and two strength training sessions. One of these cardio sessions should be high-intensity interval training (HIIT). Look at chapter 7 to see some of your top exercises. It's less about how much time you're in the gym and more about the quality of time you spend while exercising. You can get a quality workout for just 20 minutes if you're doing the right exercises in the right way. Use this QR code to connect to my fitness app that will provide you with over a hundred instructional videos to get your fitness game on point:

THE 50s

The older you get, the more your body starts to remind you that it's been in service for quite a while and things are starting to slow down a little. Your 50s are no longer regarded as a decade where you're considered "old"; 50 really is the new 40 in many ways. But for that to truly manifest, you need to be aware of what nature typically has in store for many of us during this decade and what you can do about it to soften or slow the impact.

Body Changes

Decreased bone density

Heart weakening

Joint thinning

Muscle loss

Perimenopause/
menopause

Skin changes

Weight gain

DECREASED BONE DENSITY

According to the American Academy of Orthopaedic Surgeons, most people will reach their peak bone mass somewhere between the ages of 25 and 30. Once this peak is reached, bone mass stays consistent for some time, then slowly starts to diminish. As we age, the rate of bone thinning will increase if nothing is done to stop it or slow it down. At the microscopic level, our bones are in a constant state of being created and destroyed. Bone is laid down and bone is resorbed. As we grow older, however, the laying down process doesn't keep up with the resorption process, so the bones become progressively thinner. If you add in other risk factors such as smoking, inadequate calcium or vitamin D intake, lack of weight-bearing exercise, and a disrupted hormonal environment (low estrogen in women and low testosterone in men), bone density decline is accelerated.

Fix It

At this stage of life, it's important to get ahead before you fall behind. The two most important things you can do to keep your bones healthy are exercising and consuming enough calcium. Choose weight-bearing exercises that have an impact on the body's physical skeleton, such as brisk walking, jogging or running, stair climbing, dancing, using weight machines, resistance bands, and free weights, and doing bodyweight workouts (push-ups, pull-ups, jumping jacks). Make sure you're getting enough calcium, that all-important mineral that keeps your bones strong. Both men and women should consume at least 1,000 mg of calcium each day. Vitamin D intake is also critical in helping the body absorb the calcium and phosphorus that are stored in our bones and make them stronger and more durable. If you are a smoker, stop. If you are not a smoker, don't start. Smoking can increase your risk for weakening bones. Lastly, limit your alcohol consumption. If you drink at all, drink only in moderation. Excessive alcohol consumption can cause harm to many of your organs, including the liver, brain, and bones.

A special X-ray for your bones, called a DEXA scan, is used to test for osteoporosis (or thinning of the bones). It measures the strength of your bones and lets your doctor know your risk for osteoporosis and fractures. This screening scan is typically recommended for women 65 and older; however, some women who are at an increased risk for osteoporosis might be advised to have a scan as early as age 50. This is a decision you should make in consultation with your doctor.

HEART WEAKENING

The heart is the most important muscle in the body, and just like other muscles, it can weaken over time if it's not exercised properly. The heart is comprised of four chambers: the right and left atria, which sit atop the right and left ventricles. The left ventricle is responsible for pumping oxygen-rich blood through the aorta and out to the rest of the body. Every minute, the heart pumps approximately 5 liters of blood while you are at rest. When you are exercising, that rate increases three to four times. As we become less active with age, the heart muscle behaves like other muscles and the reduced activity causes it to stiffen. This is problematic because a stiffer heart can't open or expand as well, which means there's less blood entering the left ventricle and thus less blood pumping out to the rest of the body. When you combine left ventricular stiffness and the stiffness of the arteries leading to high blood pressure, this now sets the stage for overall cardiovascular decline and conditions such as congestive heart failure (CHF). In the case of heart failure, the heart isn't pumping blood efficiently enough, leading to a backup of fluid in the lungs (because the lungs and heart are connected in sequence) and difficulty breathing.

Fix It

The answer to strengthening your heart is exercise, just like it would be for a thin and weak biceps or chest muscle. A study published in the journal *Circulation: Cardiovascular Imaging*[3] found that participants who had been only recreational runners experienced not only an increase in the size of the left ventricle but also improved overall function when put on an 18-week training regimen. The study also found that blood pressure was lowered and oxygen consumption (VO_2 max) increased while working out. All of these are desirable changes that can help reverse some of the effects of an aging and weakening heart. Exercise at different intensities to start making improvements.

1. Participate in recreational activities such as playing tennis, basketball, pickleball, racquetball, cycling, or brisk walking.
2. Exercise at moderate intensity for some of your workout sessions. You should be physically challenged by the workout but still be able to hold a conversation.
3. High-intensity interval training (HIIT) can help. Alternate intense exertion with lower exertion or rest. For example, walk or run at high intensity for a couple of minutes, then slow down to a casual pace for a couple of minutes before revving it up again. Do this for 15 to 20 minutes a session.

JOINT THINNING

Our ability to move fluidly and without pain depends on many factors, but our joints and muscles are two of the biggest players. Joints are those parts of the body where the bones come together in close proximity but don't have direct contact with each other (shoulder, knees, hips, ankles, etc.). The joints are protected by soft cartilage that cushions the ends of the bones, a fluid in the space between the bones that lubricates it (synovial fluid), and a membrane around the outside of the joint that keeps the fluid inside and protects the joint space. Unfortunately, as we age, the amount of synovial fluid decreases, and when we've lost too much fluid, the joint space narrows and there's less cushioning and ability for our bones to freely glide during movement without difficulty. This loss of synovial fluid is compounded by other changes, such as the cartilage at the end of the bones becoming thinner and the ligaments around the joint shortening and losing some of their flexibility. These changes cause the joint to become stiffer and less flexible, thus decreasing the range of motion you can achieve at the joint. Think about being able to fully bend into a squat position, but as your knee joint gets stiffer and more painful with movement, you can only go halfway down. This is what many begin to experience with aging joints, and when the joint cartilage continues to deteriorate and the underlying bone mass breaks down, this leads to the painful and physically restrictive condition called osteoarthritis.

Fix It

All of us will experience some level of joint changes as we age, but the amount and degree of these changes can be lessened if we take some preventive measures. Joints are made to be moved, and when they aren't moved properly and regularly, things become less functional. Here are a few things you can do to help avoid joint difficulties.

1. Exercise frequently.
2. Select comfortable and supportive footwear.
3. Eat a healthy diet rich in fruits, vegetables, fish, nuts, and beans and low in saturated fats.
4. Don't smoke or quit smoking.

5. Lose weight, because being overweight puts more pressure on the joints, which leads to deterioration.

MUSCLE LOSS

Muscle mass is for more than just show and bragging rights on the beach. It is critical to how we move, how we function, and for our overall health. It's much easier to build muscle in our younger years simply because we tend to have higher protein levels and our physical activity levels tend to be higher and more suitable to what's needed to grow muscle. However, as we get older, our dietary and physical activity habits change, and these changes do not favor muscle maintenance or growth. In fact, it becomes even more critical as we age to become more intentional about our protein intake. Experts suggest that we need even more protein than when we're young to help maintain our muscle mass; however, we tend to start eating less and becoming more sedentary, a combination that increases the risk of deteriorating muscle mass.

Fix It

Reversing muscle loss that's a result of aging and decreased physical activity is much easier than you might think. It doesn't require a lot of time, rather just a reasonable strategy, dedication, and consistency. It's always prudent to consult your doctor first, but here are ways to maintain or improve your muscle mass during this decade.

1. **Resistance training.** Whether it's using free weights or resistance bands, establish a consistent strength training routine that you do two to three times per week for at least 30 minutes each session.

2. **Consume protein.** Protein contains amino acids, which are the building blocks of muscle. You need sufficient amounts of protein for your muscles to grow. There are plenty of healthy animal and nonanimal sources of protein (fish, chicken, beef, beans, legumes, yogurt, chia seeds) you can add to your daily diet that will help create a better muscle-building environment. Try to consume protein-rich foods within an hour after your workout to help with muscle repair and growth.

3. **Vitamin D.** Vitamin D is not only important in helping the body absorb and retain calcium and phosphorus to build strong bone, but it's also involved in the synthesis of protein as well as increasing the size of muscle cells and muscle mass. Make sure your vitamin D levels are adequate; if they aren't, add more vitamin D–containing foods or consider taking supplements. Your healthcare provider can administer a simple blood test to help assess your vitamin D levels.

4. **Increase your omega-3s.** Omega-3 fatty acids can do more than improve brain function and protect your heart. Studies have suggested that they can contribute to muscle growth because of their anti-inflammatory properties. It's believed that omega-3s play a role in muscle protein synthesis, reducing post-workout muscle soreness, improving workout quality, and slowing muscle loss due to aging. Omega-3s can be found in many foods, including fish such as mackerel and salmon, flaxseed, chia seeds, soybeans, and nuts. You can also get quality omega-3 supplements in capsule or liquid form.

5. **Get more sleep.** One of the most important parts of muscle building is muscle recovery. Proper nutrition is a critical part of recovery, but so is getting the appropriate amount of sleep. When we sleep, our body releases human growth hormone, which can help build muscles and keep the stress hormone cortisol in check. Inadequate sleep can

also lead to a decrease in muscle-building testosterone. How much sleep do you need? There is no one answer for everyone, but most sleep experts recommend at least 7 to 9 hours of sleep per night.

PERIMENOPAUSE/MENOPAUSE

Perimenopause is the time when a woman is transitioning into menopause. This transition typically begins between the ages of 45 and 55 and usually lasts about 7 years, but for some women it can go for as long as 14 years. During perimenopause, the ovaries are still making estrogen but are gradually making less. When the ovaries stop releasing estrogen and the menstrual cycles stop, a woman is in full menopause. Many women start experiencing symptoms (hot flashes, racing heart, sweating, vaginal dryness, sore breasts, sleeping difficulty, emotional changes, dry skin) during perimenopause that might increase in frequency and intensity during menopause. Menopause is a biological inevitability, and it comes at different times and in different ways for all women. Being aware of your body and your symptoms can inform the steps you take to make this a less challenging time in your life.

Fix It

You can't stop or avoid menopause; however, you can treat or limit the severity of some of the symptoms you experience. It's important to remember that many of these symptoms will go away over time, but if they are causing problems, there's no reason you can't try to mitigate their impact now. Not all treatments work the same for everyone, and they should be taken under the supervision or in consultation with your physician. Some of them include hormone replacement therapy (HRT); nonhormone medications such as paroxetine, gabapentin, and clonidine; and selective estrogen receptor modulators (SERMS).

There are also many herbal supplements that have been promoted and reported as being beneficial for certain symptoms. Read about these treatments carefully, and make sure you get the advice of a healthcare professional before starting them.

SKIN CHANGES

Our skin is one of the first places we start to see the effects of aging. These age-related skin changes, while not necessarily desirable, are still considered to be healthy changes because they are part of the normal process of getting older. Thinning, wrinkling, and sagging will happen to everyone who lives long enough to experience them. You will encounter areas of broken blood vessels, age spots, and dry patches. The most critical unhealthy skin change that can be experienced is skin cancer, which is why limiting exposure to the sun from an early age and wearing adequate sunscreen is essential starting in childhood. Skin cancer caused by excessive sun exposure is not a condition that develops overnight. Rather, years of poor skin protection can cause microdamage to the skin cells, and this damage accumulates and multiplies in its danger until the changes become cancerous. Regular skin self-checks are important. You can read more about these self-exams in chapter 9. There is plenty you can do to protect your skin and keep it looking younger without resorting to plastic surgery or invasive dermatologic procedures. These might help in some cases, but they can be expensive, and if done too often or by an unaccredited practitioner, they can create even more damage and in some cases death. Try some of the natural fixes below to keep your skin tight and glowing.

Fix It

There are a lot of remedies besides surgery and other medical procedures that you can do to keep your skin in the best condition possible. Regardless of how good your skin care is, age will eventually take its toll, but you can reduce the severity with some simple, proactive steps.

1. **Limit sun exposure/use sunscreen.** Avoid intense sun exposure for prolonged periods of time. Wear protective clothing and eyewear, making sure you cover the less obvious areas like the back of the neck, eyes, ears, and back of the arms and legs. Use a broad-spectrum sunscreen of at least SPF 30 and apply it generously over all areas that will be exposed to the sun. Typically, a quantity that can fill a shot glass is sufficient. Reapply every 2 hours or even more frequently if you are swimming or sweating.

2. **Use moisturizer regularly.** Applying moisturizer when the skin is slightly damp can be advantageous as it helps trap the water that can be absorbed by the skin. Your skin can get dry in various climate conditions, so don't be afraid to moisturize twice a day.

3. **Use gentle skin products.** Make sure you use products that are neutral and pH-balanced. Avoid using perfumed soaps and taking long, hot showers. Bathe in warm water, making sure you use mild cleansers that won't irritate your skin. Wash gently and be careful not to scrub too hard. If you are using an exfoliant, make sure it's not so harsh that it leaves your skin raw and removes more than just the dry outer skin cells.

4. **Avoid sunlamps and tanning beds.** These machines can be extremely harmful to your skin. While you might like the appearance of being tan, tanning beds emit the same harmful UV radiation as the sun and can do as much damage if not more depending on the machine's strength and amount of time you're exposed to it. Sunlamps have been used to treat many conditions, such as seasonal affective disorder (SAD), vitamin D deficiency, and mood swings. However, they should only be used after

consulting with your doctor to determine what's safe for you.

5. **Avoid tobacco smoke.** Smoking tobacco and being exposed to it in high quantities can accelerate aging and damage your skin. Besides the dramatic cancer risk it poses, smoking changes not just the skin but your teeth and hair in ways that make you look much older. Smoking causes the skin to be chronically deprived of oxygen and nutrients, thus making it appear pale, loose, and wrinkled, especially around the mouth and eyes.

WEIGHT GAIN

People gain weight at different rates and at different times in their life. Researchers looked at data from more than 13,000 people in the National Health and Nutrition Examination Survey and published their findings in the *Journal of Obesity*.[4] They wanted to determine in which decades of their lives people put on the most pounds. The study found that on average, adults gained approximately 9.5 pounds during their 50s. Women, however, gained more than men, 13 pounds compared to 9 pounds for men. Researchers found that for each successive decade beginning when a person is in their 30s, weight gain decreased. While weight gain during this decade might not be as much as in others, it's still important to maintain a healthy weight to avoid health complications such as diabetes, heart disease, and high blood pressure. Being overweight in conjunction with other factors such as aging and being more sedentary can create an environment of health challenges.

Fix It

Build a successful weight management program that involves both a specific nutrition plan as well as an exercise regimen.

There are many weight-loss strategies that have proven effective, but the most important thing is that you choose a plan that will work for you. Make sure the food on your plan is affordable, accessible, meets your taste preferences, and that your eating strategy (low carbs, intermittent fasting, modified keto) is one you can do consistently for a long period of time. Your exercise regimen should have certain elements. You should exercise a minimum of three times a week. Your workouts should include both strength training and cardiovascular exercises. It's less about how much time you're in the gym and more about the quality of time you spend while exercising. You can get a great quality workout in just 20 minutes if you're doing the right exercises in the right way. Use the QR code below to connect with my fitness app. It will provide you with over a hundred instructional videos that can help you get your fitness game on point.

THE 60s

Your body has undergone a lot of changes since you were in your 20s, 30s, and 40s. This doesn't mean that all of these changes are bad. Our bodies age naturally. We are not machines or robots made from durable metals. We are made of water, tissues, bones, and cartilage, which means that over time our body parts are going to start showing some wear and tear. We do, however, have significant control over how well our bodies age and how long we can keep them functioning at a high level. Gaining and exerting that control effectively starts with being prepared and aware of what changes might come and what you can do to prevent them or limit their impact. In the list below, you will find some of the most common physical changes you are likely to experience during this decade and beyond. Familiarize yourself with some of these conditions and the potential proactive steps you can take to reduce their impact on your health. You can have plenty of great years to live by taking some initiative and making the most of the opportunities that life has to offer.

Body Changes

Decreased bone density

Brain shrinkage (cognitive decline)

Decreased flexibility

Heart dysfunction

Joint deterioration

Diminished lung capacity

Muscle loss

Skin changes (age spots, bruising, deep wrinkling)

DECREASED BONE DENSITY

While most people will reach their peak bone mass somewhere between the ages of 25 and 30 and maintain it at that level for a period of time, bone density starts to slowly diminish with the rate increasing as we get older. At the microscopic level, our bones are in a constant state of being created and destroyed. Bone is laid down and bone is resorbed. As we grow older, however, the laying down process doesn't keep up with the resorption process, so the bones become progressively thinner. If you add other risk factors such as smoking, inadequate calcium or vitamin D intake, lack of weight-bearing exercise, and a disrupted hormonal environment (low estrogen in women and low testosterone in men), bone density decline is accelerated. This is a decade where bone health is critical as the risk for falls and bone fractures is dramatically increased. Broken bones, especially in the lower part of the body, can be painful and lead to physical disability, but even more concerning is they can also lead to death. Hip fractures are more likely to occur in those aged 65 or older, and some estimates reveal that one in three adults aged 50 and over die within 12 months of suffering a hip fracture. It's important to remember that poor bone health doesn't just mean a curved spine and stooped posture, but it can unfortunately lead to all types of complications that can eventually be life-ending.

Fix It

Just because your bones might not be in the best of health, it doesn't mean there's nothing you can do about it. You still have the opportunity to increase your bone density through simple measures such as exercising and consuming adequate amounts of calcium. Choose weight-bearing exercises that have an impact on the body's physical skeleton, such as brisk walking, jogging or running, stair climbing, dancing, and using weight machines, resistance bands, bodyweight workouts (push-ups, pull-ups, jumping jacks), and free weights. Make sure you're getting enough calcium, that all-important mineral that keeps your bones strong. Both men and women should consume at least 1,000 mg of calcium each day. Vitamin D is also critical in helping the body absorb the calcium and phosphorus that are stored in our bones and makes them stronger and more durable. Avoid smoking and limit your alcohol intake. There are also medications that help improve your bone density, prevent bone loss, and lower the risk of broken bones. You can discuss with your healthcare provider if these are an option you should consider.

A special X-ray for your bones, called a DEXA scan, is used to test for osteoporosis or thinning of the bones. It measures the strength of your bones and lets your doctor know your risk for osteoporosis and fractures. This screening scan is typically recommended for women 65 and older; however, some women who are at an increased risk for osteoporosis might be advised to have a scan as early as age 50. This is a decision you should make in consultation with your doctor.

BRAIN SHRINKAGE (COGNITIVE DECLINE)

The brain stops growing in size by early adolescence, but it's not until the mid- to late 20s when the brain finishes developing and maturing. After the age of 40, the volume of the brain and/or its weight declines at a rate of approximately 5 percent per decade. This rate of shrinkage/decline might accelerate for some if they experience conditions such as stroke, infection, injury, or Huntington's disease. This decline might also increase for those over the age of 70 even if they are otherwise healthy. While there can be a variety of changes that correspond to this brain atrophy, the most widely seen and studied cognitive change is that of memory. All of us at a certain age will start experiencing memory challenges, whether it's forgetting where we put the car keys or recalling the name of an old school mate. This type of memory loss is considered normal and different from memory loss due to diseases such as dementia or Alzheimer's.

Fix It

The simple fact of life is that the brain shrinks as we age and there's nothing that can be done to reverse that. However, there are things we can do to keep our brain as young and functional as possible.

1. **Diet counts.** Good nutrition can help all parts of your body, including the brain. Numerous sources have shown that a Mediterranean-style diet that focuses on fruits, vegetables, nuts, fish, legumes, and unsaturated oils can reduce your chances of developing cognitive decline and dementia.

2. **Mental stimulation.** Brain-powered activities such as crossword puzzles, word games, and reading can prompt the formation of new connections between nerve cells. This helps develop what's called neurological plasticity,

in which the brain is consistently rewiring itself and modifying its connections, thus building up a functional reserve that can diminish the impact of future cell loss. Research has also shown that engaging in relationships with others and being part of a community where there's a connection and a feeling of belonging can help prevent or slow cognitive decline.

3. **Lower your cholesterol.** High levels of the low-density lipoprotein (LDL) cholesterol have been associated with an increased risk of dementia, though the exact mechanism of how cholesterol plays a role hasn't been fully worked out. Improving your diet, exercising regularly, avoiding tobacco, losing weight, and taking certain medications (if necessary) can all help reduce your LDL cholesterol level.

4. **Exercise.** The benefits of exercise at all ages are enormous and life-changing. Exercise spurs the development of new nerve cells and increases the connections between brain cells. These changes can make the brain more adaptive, efficient, and elastic, which can help maintain or improve functioning. Exercise can also help lower LDL cholesterol levels, increase your high-density lipoprotein (HDL) levels, and lower blood pressure, two other factors that can increase your risk for dementia and mental decline.

5. **Avoid tobacco/Limit alcohol intake.** This is a no-brainer (pun intended). Avoid all forms of tobacco. Don't abuse alcohol. If you're going to drink, limit it to no more than two drinks a day for men and one for women.

DECREASED FLEXIBILITY

This is the decade where you might become increasingly aware of your loss of flexibility. Years of being physically inactive, overweight, or suffering from movement-limiting conditions such as arthritis could have led to decreased muscle strength, joint range of motion, and soft tissue elasticity. Retirement can also be a big change in your lifestyle as some retirees become less active without the daily need to go to work and spend more of their time being sedentary. Your body's various joints need to be regularly put through a full range of motions, your muscles need to be challenged, and your soft tissues need to be frequently stretched. A limber and supple body means a lower risk of injury and increased physical abilities that allow you to continue being active and satisfied.

Fix It

Foam rollers, which might look very simple and unsophisticated, can be extremely helpful in helping to stretch out those cranky soft tissues. Muscles are covered by fascia, a thin layer of connective tissue that also embeds itself throughout the muscle fibers. Both the muscles and the fascia can tighten as you age or if you're injured. Besides using a foam roller, there are other techniques and devices that can help you achieve myofascial release and regain flexibility. Roll the targeted areas up and down over the foam roller several times a week for just a few minutes. Regular stretching is also important and should be done several times a week. It doesn't require a lot of time, but consistency is key. Yoga is one of the most popular methods of stretching, but there are also entire classes online and in person that focus on increasing strength and flexibility through stretching. Lastly, participating in sports is still possible, especially things like pickleball, which has become wildly popular and can be played by people of all ages and various levels of fitness. Find sports like this or activities (dancing, swimming, exercising to music) that you enjoy and do it consistently to get the best results and most satisfaction.

HEART DYSFUNCTION

According to the National Institute on Aging, people aged 65 and older are much more likely than younger people to develop coronary artery disease (disease of the blood vessels that feed the heart muscles), suffer a heart attack, have a stroke, or experience heart failure (inadequate heart pumping). Our heart muscles, particularly those in the left ventricle chamber, become stiffer with age as do our blood vessels, thus preventing the heart from pumping as much blood per beat as it used to. Our hearts can't beat as fast during physical activity or during stressful times. Fatty deposits might build up in the walls of our arteries, and when this buildup is great enough, it can cause myriad problems. The electrical system that powers the heart can also show signs of aging that manifest as an irregular heartbeat. The valves that allow the blood inside the heart to pass from one chamber to another can become thicker and stiffen with age, and this can limit the amount of blood that is pumped out of the heart as well as cause leaks from one chamber to another, causing fluid to back up into the lungs and/or body (swollen abdomen, feet, and legs).

Fix It

Age-related changes of the heart can be prevented, slowed, or treated in many ways. Regular exercise; a diet low in saturated fats, salt, and added sugars; maintaining a healthy weight; quitting smoking or avoiding tobacco smoke; reducing stress; limiting alcohol intake; and properly managing chronic medical conditions such as diabetes and high blood pressure can help keep your heart strong, healthy, and young.

JOINT DETERIORATION

Our ability to move fluidly and without pain depends on many factors, but our joints and muscles are two of the biggest players. Joints are the parts of the body where bones come together in close proximity but don't directly contact each other. The joints are protected by soft cartilage that cushions the ends of the bones, a fluid in the space between the bones that lubricates it called synovial fluid, and a membrane around the outside of the joint that keeps the fluid inside and protects the joint space. Unfortunately, as we age, the amount of synovial fluid decreases, and when too much fluid is lost, the joint space narrows and there's less cushioning and ability for our bones to freely glide during movement. This loss of synovial fluid is compounded by other changes, such as the cartilage at the end of the bones becoming thinner and the ligaments around the joint shortening and losing some of their flexibility. These changes cause the joint to become stiffer and less flexible thus decreasing range of motion. Think about your knees and imagine being able to fully bend into a squat position. When your joints get stiffer and more painful with movement, you can't bend all the way down, rather you can only go maybe halfway down or less. This is what many begin to experience with aging joints, and when the conditions continue to deteriorate even further, a state of disrepair is reached called osteoarthritis.

Fix It

All of us will experience some level of joint changes as we age, but the amount and degree of these changes can be lessened if we take some preventive measures. Many of the joint changes experienced are mainly because of a lack of movement. Joints are designed to move, and when they aren't exercised properly and regularly, they start to lose functionality. Here are a few things you can do to help avoid joint difficulties.

1. Exercise frequently.
2. Select comfortable and supportive footwear.
3. Eat a healthy diet rich in fruits, vegetables, fish, nuts, and beans and low in saturated fats.
4. Don't smoke or quit smoking.
5. Lose weight.

DIMINISHED LUNG CAPACITY

Lungs tend to reach maturity between the ages of 20 to 25. However, after about the age of 35, it's normal for lung function to gradually decline. The diaphragm, a thin, dome-shaped muscle that sits just below the lungs and heart, is responsible for our ability to breathe. When it contracts and flattens during inhalation, the chest cavity enlarges, creating a vacuum that pulls air into the lungs. During exhalation, the diaphragm muscle relaxes and returns to its domelike shape, forcing air out of the lungs. Like any other muscle in the body, it can get weaker with age. The condition of our lung tissue also is important for normal breathing. Just like our skin loses elasticity and begins to sag as we age, the lung tissue that keeps our airways open can lose its elasticity, causing the lungs to become smaller and reducing their ability to fully expand. When our airways can't expand maximally, the amount of air our lungs inhale and exhale becomes diminished. These changes can result in breathing becoming more difficult and a decline in cardiovascular endurance. Physical activities that you have been doing for years suddenly exhaust you faster or your performance declines because of fatigue. It's important to separate the loss of lung capacity and function due to aging from that caused by diseases such as fibrosis, pneumonia, congestive heart failure, and cancer. If you're experiencing sudden breathing difficulties or otherwise unexplained shortness of breath, see your doctor immediately for a full examination.

Fix It

All of us will experience age-related lung decline, but how much and how quickly it declines can potentially be controlled by some actions we take and choices we make.

1. **Don't smoke.** The data supporting this has been around a long time and is overwhelming.
2. **Exercise.** Being physically active at any age helps keep your lungs healthy.
3. **High indoor air quality.** Most people spend 90 percent of their time indoors. The air quality inside is just as important as the air quality outside. In some cases, indoor air can be more polluted than outdoor. Chemicals at home or the workplace, secondhand smoke, and mold are just some of the pollutants that can damage our lungs. Some ways to keep the air clean in your house: Control the humidity to avoid growth of mold and dust mites; avoid smoking indoors; use high-efficiency particulate air (HEPA) filters in an air purifier; ventilate by opening windows and doors (weather permitting); regularly clean carpets and furniture; consider adding houseplants (peace lilies, snake plants, spider plants, etc.) to your indoor spaces as they can help remove toxins from the air.
4. **Monitor outdoor air quality.** There are a lot of environmental pollutants contaminating air quality. Minimize the time you spend outdoors when pollution is high. You can even monitor the air quality index (AQI) right from your smartphone via various apps. Airnow.gov is a popular site/app that's being widely used for this purpose.
5. **Regular check-ups.** Your lungs, just like your heart and blood pressure, should be checked regularly by a healthcare provider. Changes and symptoms that you might notice can be recognized by your healthcare professional.

MUSCLE LOSS

Muscle size and strength are important contributors to good health and functionality, especially as we age and reach a time in life when our bodies don't seem as responsive and capable as in previous years. Muscles are critical to how we move, how we function, and our overall health. It's much easier to build muscle in our younger years, but as we get older, more protein and resistance exercises are musts to improve or maintain muscle mass and strength. It's important not to give up and resign yourself to the idea that as we age we are not meant to have muscles and growing weaker should be expected. We tend to get weaker as we age, because our nutrition isn't optimal and our physical activities are diminished and not focused on muscle building and preservation.

Fix It

Reversing muscle loss that's due to aging and decreased physical activity is much easier than you might think. It doesn't require a lot of time, just a reasonable strategy, dedication, and consistency. Consult your healthcare provider before starting a new workout regimen.

Here are some ways to maintain or improve your muscle mass during this decade.

1. **Resistance training.** Whether it's using free weights or resistance bands, establish a consistent strength training routine that you do two to three times per week for at least 30 minutes each session.
2. **Consume protein.** Protein contains amino acids, which are the building blocks of muscle. You need protein for your muscles to grow and heal. There are plenty of healthy animal and nonanimal sources of protein (fish, chicken, beef, beans, legumes, yogurt, chia seeds) you can add

to your daily diet that will help create a better muscle-building environment. Try to consume protein-rich foods within an hour after your workout to help with muscle repair and growth.

3. **Vitamin D.** Vitamin D is not only important in helping the body absorb and retain calcium and phosphorus to build strong bone, but it's also involved in the synthesis of protein as well as increasing the size of muscle cells and muscle mass. Make sure your vitamin D levels are adequate; if they aren't, add more vitamin D–containing foods or consider taking supplements. Your healthcare provider can administer a simple blood test that can help assess your levels.

4. **Increase your omega-3s.** Omega-3 fatty acids can do more than improve brain function and protect your heart. Studies have suggested that they can contribute to muscle growth because of their anti-inflammatory properties. It's believed that omega-3s play a role in muscle protein synthesis, reducing post-workout muscle soreness, improving workout quality, and slowing muscle loss due to aging. Omega-3s can be found in many foods, including fish such as mackerel and salmon, flaxseed, chia seeds, soybeans, and nuts. You can also get quality omega-3 supplements in a capsule or liquid form.

5. **Get more sleep.** One of the most important parts of muscle building is muscle recovery. Proper nutrition is a critical part of recovery, but so is getting the appropriate amount of sleep. When we sleep, our body releases human growth hormone, which can help muscles grow and keep the stress hormone cortisol in check. Inadequate sleep can also lead to a decrease in muscle-building testosterone. How much sleep do you need? There is no one answer for everyone, but most sleep experts recommend at least 7 to 9 hours of sleep per night.

SKIN CHANGES

Our skin is one of the first places we start to see the effects of aging. These age-related skin changes, while not necessarily desirable, are still considered to be healthy changes because they are part of the normal process of getting older. Thinning, wrinkling, and sagging skin will happen to everyone who lives long enough to experience them. You will encounter areas of broken blood vessels, age spots, and dry patches. The most critical unhealthy skin change that can be experienced is skin cancer, which is why limiting exposure to the sun from an early age and wearing adequate sunscreen are essential starting in childhood. Skin cancer caused by excessive sun exposure is not a condition that develops overnight. Rather, years of poor skin protection can cause microdamage to the skin cells, and this damage accumulates and multiplies in its danger until the changes become cancerous. Regular skin self-checks are important. You can read more about these self-exams in chapter 9. There is plenty you can do to protect your skin and keep it looking younger without resorting to plastic surgery or invasive dermatologic procedures. These procedures might help in some cases, but they can be expensive and if done too often or by an unaccredited practitioner, they can create even more damage and in some cases death. Try some of the natural fixes below to keep your skin wrinkle-free and glowing.

Fix It

The effects that age and environmental stimuli can have on your skin can sometimes be reversed to some degree or minimized. There are simple, proactive steps that can make a difference.

1. **Limit sun exposure/use sunscreen.** Avoid intense sun exposure for prolonged periods of time. Wear protective clothing and eyewear, making sure to cover the less

obvious spots like the back of the neck, eyes, ears, and back of the arms and legs. Use a broad-spectrum sunscreen of at least SPF 30 and apply generously over all areas that will be exposed to the sun. Typically, a quantity that can fill a shot glass is sufficient. Reapply every 2 hours or more frequently if you are swimming or sweating.

2. **Use moisturizer regularly.** Applying moisturizer when the skin is slightly damp can be advantageous as it helps trap moisture that can be absorbed by the skin. If your skin gets dry in various climate conditions, don't be afraid to moisturize twice a day.

3. **Use gentle skin products.** Make sure to use products that are neutral and pH-balanced. Avoid using perfumed soaps and taking long, hot showers. Bathe in warm water, making sure to use mild cleansers that won't irritate your skin. Wash gently and don't scrub too hard. If you are using an exfoliant, make sure it's not so harsh that it leaves your skin raw and removes more than just the dry outer skin cells.

4. **Avoid sunlamps and tanning beds.** These machines can be extremely harmful to your skin. While you might like the experience of being tan, tanning beds emit the same harmful UV radiation as the sun and can do as much damage if not more, depending on the machine's strength and amount of time you're exposed to it. Sunlamps have been used to treat many conditions, such as seasonal affective disorder (SAD), vitamin D deficiency, and mood swings. However, they should only be used after consulting your doctor and determining what's safe for you.

5. **Avoid tobacco smoke.** Smoking tobacco and being exposed to it in high quantities can accelerate aging and damage your skin. Besides the dramatic cancer risk it

poses, smoking changes not just the skin but your teeth and hair in ways that make you look much older. Smoking causes the skin to be chronically deprived of oxygen and nutrients, thus making the skin appear pale, loose, and wrinkled, especially around the mouth and eyes.

9

YOUR TOP MEDICAL TESTS

The saying "An ounce of prevention is worth a pound of cure" couldn't be truer when considering the aging process and how it sometimes feels like we're navigating a minefield. Some of the most important preventive measures to avoid serious illnesses come in the form of screening tests, where doctors can do a quick analysis of blood work or scans of particular body parts to make sure all is intact, and if not, sound the alarm for either more tests or early treatment. Screening tests are often painless, fast, and inexpensive, but millions of people don't get them because they either don't know about them, don't understand them, or simply put them off and never get around to doing them.

To potentially avoid unnecessary illness and suffering, talk to your healthcare provider about the tests that are most relevant to you—it could help you live not just a longer life but one of a much better quality. In this chapter, you will find explanations of the tests that are most important for your decade of life. Look at this as your preventive road map to better and sustained good health.

Each decade section lists the top 10 tests, but talk to your doctor about other tests that should be on your list based on your and your relatives' medical history and risk factors for certain conditions. Also, in some cases there are more than 10 tests listed in the table because some of the tests are exclusively for women (breast and mammograms) and others for men (prostate PSA and digital rectal exam).

NUMBERS TO KNOW

30S	40S	50S	60S
Blood Glucose Levels	Blood Glucose Levels	Blood Glucose Levels	Blood Glucose Levels
Blood Pressure	Blood Pressure	Blood Pressure	Blood Pressure
Cholesterol	Breast Exam/ Mammogram	Bone Density	Bone Density
Dental Exam/ Cleaning	Colorectal Screening	Breast Exam/ Mammogram	Breast Exam/ Mammogram
Depression/ Anxiety/ PTSD	Dental Exam/ Cleaning	Cholesterol	Cholesterol
Eye Exam	Eye Exam	Colorectal	Colorectal
Pelvic Exam/ Pap Smear/HPV	Pelvic Exam (women)	Dental Exam/ Cleaning	Dental Exam/ Cleaning
Sexually Transmitted Infections (STI)	PSA/Digital Rectal Exam (men)	Eye Exam	Eye Exam
Skin Check	Sexually Transmitted Infections (STI)	Pelvic Exam (women)	Hearing
Urinalysis	Skin Check	PSA/Digital Rectal Exam (men)	Pelvic Exam (women)
		Sexually Transmitted Infections (STI)	PSA/Digital Rectal Exam (men)
		Skin Check	Sexually Transmitted Infections (STI)
			Skin Check

The purpose of these lists is to help you better understand the related tests and provide context to have a more thorough conversation with your doctor about your specific needs. For example, you might have chronic anemia, so your doctor might order blood tests to monitor your condition more effectively. Or you might have a personal or family history of breast cancer or prostate cancer, and your doctor might order different tests to screen for disease or to monitor your condition if you've already been diagnosed. The lists here are just guidelines; your physician can advise you on what you need.

30S

It's true that the older we get, the more our body seems to become off-kilter and start breaking down. Though testing becomes more imperative the older we get, it doesn't mean we shouldn't start as early as our 30s. Become aware of your health, and take proactive measures that will be important for your health now and in the future as well. The tests listed for your decade can help you keep proper inventory of your health and help raise early warning signs should something be amiss.

40S

Regardless of how busy your life is or how good you might look and feel, getting the proper screening tests on a regular basis is essential to staying healthy and disease-free for as long as possible. The older we get, the greater the risk of developing acute and chronic medical conditions. The aim of this chapter is to help you focus on the tests that can keep you informed and proactive on your health journey.

50S

This is the decade where the lifestyle decisions and behaviors you've made over the last 49 years start manifesting in real ways, some that are less desirable than others. This, however, doesn't mean you can't right the ship if it's a little off course. There are plenty more healthy and happy years in your future, but it requires you to take your health seriously and start making better decisions more consistently. Don't be afraid to take stock of where you are as this will arm you with the information you need to take the necessary steps to improve and monitor your health.

60s+

This decade and the ones that follow can provide plenty of opportunities for you to enjoy many years of good health, happiness, and high productivity. Your perspective is as critical as your physical health. These are the years where you can still make changes that will provide real and lasting benefits. By no means should you be looking into the sky thinking that the sun is setting on your life and there's nothing you can do about it. Instead, get up every morning with the positive perspective that the sun is actually rising and there can be plenty of sunrises in your future if you are determined and willing to take steps for that to happen. A good attitude, staying self-aware of your body, and getting the necessary screening tests can go a long way in keeping that sun rising and shining in your life.

BLOOD GLUCOSE LEVEL

Glucose is a type of sugar and a member of the large family of carbohydrates. It is one of the body's most important fuel sources and is extremely important when consumed in appropriate amounts and processed correctly. When the body is not able to process glucose properly, too much of it remains circulating in the blood, which can lead to problems, including damage to the kidneys, eyes, nerves, and blood vessels. When blood sugar levels remain abnormally high, this leads to diabetes.

According to the Centers for Disease Control and Prevention (CDC), 37.3 million Americans have diabetes. That's equivalent to approximately 11.3 percent of the entire population. Of these, 28.7 million have been formally diagnosed and 8.6 million are undiagnosed, living their lives with diabetes and unaware of it. There are two major types of diabetes, Type 1 and Type 2. Type 1 is less common than

Type 2, and while it can occur at any age, it's typically first diagnosed in childhood. Type 2 is the most common form of diabetes and is typically diagnosed in adults but can also be diagnosed in children.

There are different tests below that screen for blood glucose regulation. The test(s) that you specifically need is based on several factors. A full discussion with your healthcare provider can help you determine which of these tests you need and how frequently you should have them performed.

RANDOM PLASMA GLUCOSE TEST

This simple blood test is performed at any time of the day, and unlike other tests, it doesn't matter how recently you've had anything to eat or drink.

RANDOM PLASMA GLUCOSE

RESULT	RANDOM PLASMA GLUCOSE (MILLIGRAMS PER DECILITER)
Normal	Less than or 200
Diabetes	Greater than or equal to 200

FASTING PLASMA GLUCOSE TEST (FPG)

Typically performed first thing in the morning before breakfast, this blood test analyzes your blood glucose levels while fasting (not having anything to eat or drink, except water, for at least 8 hours before the test.

FASTING PLASMA GLUCOSE

RESULT	FASTING PLASMA GLUCOSE (MILLIGRAMS PER DECILITER)
Normal	Less than 100
Prediabetes	100 to 125
Diabetes	126 or higher

ORAL GLUCOSE TOLERANCE TEST (OGTT)

This is a 2-hour test that specifically checks your blood glucose levels before you drink a special sweet drink and 2 hours after you drink it. The results are an indicator of how well your body can process sugar.

ORAL GLUCOSE TOLERANCE TEST

RESULT	ORAL GLUCOSE TOLERANCE TEST (MILLIGRAMS PER DECILITER)
Normal	Less than 140
Prediabetes	140 to 199
Diabetes	200 or higher

HEMOGLOBIN A1C

This blood test measures your average blood glucose levels for the past 2 to 3 months. This gives an indication of how well or poorly your body has processed and maintained proper blood sugar levels. While the other tests are a quick snapshot of how well your body is regulating blood sugar levels, this provides a longer-term analysis.

HEMOGLOBIN A1C (HBA1C) (%)

Normal	Less than 5.6
Prediabetes	5.7 to 6.4
Diabetes	Higher than 6.5

PREDIABETES

Everyone who has elevated blood sugar levels is not necessarily diabetic. In fact, according to the CDC, 96 million people 18 years of age and older (38 percent of the US population) have what's called prediabetes, which means their blood sugar levels are higher than normal, but not so high that they are classified as having full-blown diabetes. The good news with a prediabetes diagnosis is that progression to diabetes is not inevitable. Those with prediabetes are virtually straddling the fence. They can fall completely over to the other side, or they can adopt lifestyle behavioral changes and return to normal blood sugar levels, thus avoiding the long-term damage of diabetes. Getting the proper screenings, eating your top nutrients consistently, and exercising regularly can help prevent prediabetes from converting into full-blown Type 2 diabetes.

TEST	RESULT	DIAGNOSIS
Fasting Plasma Glucose	100 to 125 milligrams per deciliter	Prediabetes
Hemoglobin A1C	5.7% to 6.4%	Prediabetes

BLOOD PRESSURE

This is a simple test that can be performed by a doctor, nurse, or health technician with a simple stethoscope and an inflatable arm cuff. There are two important numbers being measured. The upper number is the systolic number, which represents the pressure inside your arteries when your heart is beating (heart muscle contracting). The lower number is the diastolic number, which represents the pressure inside your arteries when your heart is resting between beats. If you use a machine at home or in a store, make sure you record multiple readings, and if there is an abnormality, have your blood pressure checked at your doctor's office for confirmation. Many at-home machines and in-store machines can give erroneous readings. Also, your environment, mood, posture, and behavior before taking your blood pressure can have an impact on the result, which is why confirmation needs to be made by an experienced medical professional. There is no universal recommendation for

BLOOD PRESSURE CATEGORY	SYSTOLIC MM HG (UPPER NUMBER)	AND/ OR	DIASTOLIC MM HG (LOWER NUMBER)
Normal	Less than 120	and	Less than 80
Elevated	120 to 129	and	Less than 80
High Blood Pressure (Hypertension) Stage 1	130 to 139	or	80 to 89
High Blood Pressure (Hypertension) Stage 2	140 or Higher	or	90 or Higher
Hypertensive Crisis (consult your doctor immediately	Higher than 180	and/or	Higher than 120

Source: American Heart Association

how often you should measure your blood pressure. Most experts suggest at least once every 1 to 2 years, but this, of course, changes based on several risk factors and predisposition to high blood pressure. The exact schedule is something that needs to be determined by you and your doctor to make sure your monitoring of this important number is adequate.

BONE DENSITY

Bone density screenings are performed to determine if someone has osteoporosis. This test is also referred to as a bone mass measurement or bone mineral density test. The most common test performed is called a DEXA scan (short for dual-energy X-ray absorptiometry). This machine uses X-rays to measure how many grams of calcium and other important bone minerals are concentrated in a segment of bone, thus giving an indication of the strength and density of your bones. Not all the bones need to be tested, rather a sample, which typically consists of the hip, spine, and/or forearm. The test is painless, noninvasive, and safe. It can be extremely helpful, because it can not only be used to confirm a diagnosis of osteoporosis and monitor the condition once treatment starts, but it can detect low bone density *before* a fracture occurs. A bone density test is also used to predict your chances of fracturing in the future.

There are no universally agreed-upon guidelines for who should be getting screened and how often. The US Preventive Services Task Force (USPSTF) recommendations look only at women and suggest that those 65 and older should start getting their bone mineral density measured. Their recommendation also states that women younger than 65 who are postmenopausal and have an increased risk of osteoporosis should start screening. Unfortunately, the recommendations don't address men, who might develop osteoporosis less often but are certainly vulnerable to bone loss as they age. When to start getting scanned and how often you should be scanned are decisions that need to be made in consultation with your doctor based on your medical history and risk factors. Some doctors even recommend their patients start getting scanned at age 50, depending on their risk profile and other important factors.

T-SCORE

For the sake of convention, the bone mineral density of the average healthy young adult is considered to be 0. The machine uses a mathematical formula to see how your bone density compares to this average healthy young adult. If your bones are weaker,

T-SCORE

T-SCORE	BONE DENSITY STATUS
1 or higher	Healthy
-1 to -2.5	Osteopenia (low bone mineral density, but not as severe as what is seen in osteoporosis)
-2.5 or lower	High chance of osteoporosis

Source: National Institute of Arthritis and Musculoskeletal and Skin Diseases

your T-score will be a negative number. If your bones have equal density (strength) or more, your score will be a positive number.

Every time your T-score drops by 1 point, the risk of your breaking a bone increases by 1.5 to 2 times.

Z-SCORE

Premenopausal women, men younger than 50, and children get their test results in what's called a Z-score. This score represents the difference between your bone mineral density and the bone mineral density of healthy people of the same age, ethnicity, and gender. A Z-score of -2.0 or less is an indicator of low bone density, which means you might have osteoporosis; further testing should be done and a treatment plan developed.

BREAST EXAM AND MAMMOGRAM

A clinical breast exam is performed by a healthcare professional in an exam room. They use their hands to feel for lumps or any other changes in the breast tissue that might indicate an abnormality that needs to be studied further. According to the American College of Obstetricians and Gynecologists, women aged 40 and older should have a clinical breast exam performed every year. It's also important for women to examine their own breasts since they are most familiar with their bodies and more likely to pick up on any changes. Breast self-exams (BSE) should be done once a month about 7 to 10 days after your menstrual period, which is when the breasts are the least tender and lumpy. For women who are no longer menstruating, choose the same day of the month to do the exam and do it every month. To learn how to perform a BSE, go to https://www.youtube.com/watch?v=I7wSEIOz-1k.

AGE	RECOMMENDATION
40 to 45	Optional to start screening with a mammogram every year.
45 to 54	Should get mammograms every year.
55 and older	The option to switch to a mammogram every other year or choose to continue yearly mammograms. Screening should continue as long as a woman is in good health and expected to live at least 10 more years.

Source: American Cancer Society

A mammogram is a special X-ray of the breast that takes a closer look at the tissue and overall anatomy. The US Preventive Services Task Force recommends that women between the ages of 40 and 49 should talk to their doctor or other healthcare provider about when to start and how often to get a mammogram. The benefits and risks of the test need to be considered as well as what a woman's specific risk factors are for breast cancer. For example, most experts recommend that women who have an increased risk for breast cancer should start getting mammograms in their 40s.

CHOLESTEROL

This simple blood test is part of what's called a lipid profile, which measures cholesterol as well as various other fats in the blood. This test can give your healthcare provider a lot of information about your total cholesterol, LDL (bad) cholesterol, HDL (good) cholesterol, and triglycerides. This information can paint a picture of how well you're processing fats as well as your risk profile for blood vessel and cardiovascular disease. Unless you are at high risk for cardiovascular disease or cholesterol-related disorders, the general recommendation is for adults to check their cholesterol levels every 4 to 6 years. If you have risk factors, your doctor might determine a more frequent schedule for checking your cholesterol and other fats.

	TOTAL CHOLESTEROL	LDL CHOLESTEROL	HDL CHOLESTEROL
Dangerous	240 and higher	160 and higher	Under 40 (male) Under 50 (female)
At Risk	200 to 239	100 to 159	40 to 59 (male) 50 to 59 (female)
Heart Healthy	Under 200	Under 100	60 and higher

COLORECTAL SCREENING

People who have no symptoms of colorectal cancer can undergo various screening tests to detect if cancer is present. There are two main groups of tests: stool-based and visual (structural) exams. There are five tests between the two groups that are commonly used. The three common stool-based tests are the fecal occult blood test, fecal immunochemical test, and the DNA stool test.

There are three visual exams of the colon and rectum: colonoscopy, CT colonography, and flexible sigmoidoscopy.

A colonoscopy is where a long, flexible tube (colonoscope) with a camera at the tip is inserted into the rectum. The doctor advances the colonoscope from the rectum to the large intestine up into the small intestine and can see the inside of the entire colon. If any abnormalities are seen, such as polyps, the doctor can remove the abnormal tissue and study it under a microscope to determine if it's cancerous.

CT colonography, also called virtual colonoscopy, uses special X-ray equipment to examine the large intestine. A small tube is inserted only a short distance into the rectum from which gas or air is used to inflate the colon and rectum. Once dilation has occurred, X-ray pictures are taken.

GENERAL SCREENING RECOMMENDATIONS BASED ON AGE

AGE	AVERAGE RISK*	HIGH RISK**
Under 45	No screening	Consult your physician as to your particular risk profile. Some doctors will recommend early screening.
45	Start screening	Consult your physician.
46 to 75	Continue screening (Up until 75 if you are in good health and with a life expectancy of more than 10 years. The type of screening and frequency are based on one's risk factors and medical history.)	Consult your physician.
75 to 85	Screening optional (Decision is personal and made in conjunction with healthcare provider and should be based on personal preferences, life expectancy, overall health, and prior screening history.)	Consult your physician.
Over 85	No colorectal cancer screening.	Consult your physician.

Source: American Cancer Society

*NO personal history of colorectal cancer or certain types of polyps, family history of colorectal cancer, personal history of inflammatory bowel disease such as ulcerative colitis or Crohn's, confirmed or suspected hereditary colorectal cancer syndrome, personal history of getting radiation to the abdomen or pelvic area to treat a prior cancer

**Personal history of colorectal cancer or certain types of polyps, family history of colorectal cancer, personal history of inflammatory bowel disease such as ulcerative colitis or Crohn's, confirmed or suspected hereditary colorectal cancer syndrome, personal history of getting radiation to the abdomen or pelvic area to treat a prior cancer

A flexible sigmoidoscopy uses a narrow tube with a light and tiny camera at its end inserted into the rectum and advanced only into the lower portion of the colon (large intestine). With this camera, the doctor can see inside the rectum and lower colon.

Recommendations for colorectal screening can be quite a maze. Different credible organizations have different recommendations, which are left to interpretation by the doctor along with the patient's medical history and the presence of other risk factors.

The American Cancer Society recommends that people at average risk of colorectal cancer start screening at 45 years old. Your doctor might suggest either a stool-based test or a visual imaging test or both. People are considered high risk if they have: a confirmed or suspected hereditary colorectal cancer syndrome, family history of colorectal cancer, personal history of colorectal cancer or certain types of polyps, personal history of getting radiation to the abdomen or pelvic area to treat a prior cancer, or personal history of inflammatory bowel disease.

DENTAL EXAMS/CLEANINGS

There are no hard-and-fast rules when it comes to the frequency of dental visits and examinations. Most experts recommend at least once a year, which can also include a cleaning. However, based on your dental history and needs, this schedule could be adjusted in consultation with your dentist. If you are at high risk for oral disease or actively managing a condition, your dentist might recommend more frequent visits. Regular dental visits can help prevent cavities or catch cavities at an early stage when they can be effectively treated. Missing out on the opportunity to catch cavities early can lead to more expensive and complicated treatments that can also be more painful. Seeing your dentist can also lead to diagnosing other conditions such as gum disease and even non-oral-health conditions such as diabetes. Good dental health is not just about a good smile; it's important for your overall health as well.

DEPRESSION/ANXIETY/PTSD SCREENING

Mental illness does not discriminate. It affects people of all ages, genders, races, and socioeconomic backgrounds. The recent focus of the last several years on encouraging sufferers to come forward and seek help for mental health challenges without shame or penalty has been a major paradigm shift in how mental illness is viewed, treated, and supported. There has always been an understanding within the field of medicine that many more people suffered from mental health challenges than the data suggested. Now that there is greater awareness, openness, and sensitivity, the new data is starting to more accurately resemble the true prevalence of mental illness. There are many types of mental disorders; however, three of them—anxiety disorders, depression, and post-traumatic stress disorder (PTSD)—make up approximately 30 percent of all mental illness diagnoses in the United States. The US Preventive Services Task Force recommends screening for depression and anxiety in the adult population, including pregnant and postpartum persons as well as older adults. Specifically, it's recommended that all adults between the ages of 19 and 64 be screened for anxiety disorders and all adults, including those 65 and older, be screened for major depressive disorder. There are different types of screening methods for mental health disorders, so determining which is best and the frequency with which the screening tool should be applied are decisions that should be made by you and your healthcare provider. The most important thing is that, regardless of your age or station in life, you should feel free to seek help if you think you're suffering from a mental health challenge. There is no prototype person or exact profile of someone who is either at risk or suffering from a mental health challenge. Everyone has the potential to be affected, thus being self-aware and more in tune with what's happening emotionally can hopefully prompt reaching out for help if needed.

Dr. Ian's Tips

GET OUT AND SOCIALIZE

There's a lot to be said about building and forging relationships whether they be with family or friends. Not only does it seem to be common sense that human beings thrive and fare better when they have supportive, positive relationships, but studies have shown that people who have meaningful connections and frequent interactions with family members and friends are not only healthier but live longer than those who don't engage in deeper relationships.

EYE EXAM

A complete eye exam involves other aspects beyond checking your visual acuity. Doctors want to assess the overall health of the eye as well as other measurements, such as intraocular pressure and refraction with regard to your lens. Many eye and vision-related problems don't have obvious signs or symptoms, so you may be unaware that a problem even exists. You don't want to ignore or minimize potential eye problems because early treatment can greatly increase

EYE EXAMINATION INTERVAL

PATIENT AGE (YEARS)	ASYMPTOMATIC/ LOW RISK	AT RISK*
18 to 39	At least every 2 years	At least annually, or as recommended
40 to 64	At least every 2 years	At least annually, or as recommended
65 and older	Annually	At least annually, or as recommended

Source: American Optometric Association

*Those who have a personal past medical history, family history, or lifestyle might be at higher risk and thus fall into this category. Your doctor will help you determine your risk profile.

your chances of preventing damage that can lead to vision loss. How often you get your eyes examined and which tests should be performed will depend on several factors and should be discussed with your doctor.

HEARING TEST

As we age, hearing loss becomes more likely to occur. Approximately 14 percent of people between the ages of 45 and 64 have some degree of hearing loss. For people 65 and older, this number increases to as much as 30 percent. Many experts recommend getting your hearing tested every 10 years up until the age of 50, then every 3 years after that. There are many causes for hearing loss, including excessive ear wax, ruptured ear drum, infection, bone growths/tumors, and damage to the inner ear, many of which can be treated if caught early. It's important not to dismiss hearing troubles. Get examined by your doctor and discuss causes and treatment options. A hearing test is painless and takes approximately 30 minutes. The most common one, the pure-tone hearing test, measures the softest or least audible sound you can hear at different pitches or frequencies. You may have had this test performed when you were in elementary school. The test requires you to wear headphones and raise your hand when you hear a beeping sound. Sound is measured in decibels (dB). For example, a whisper is about 20 to 30 dB, whereas shouting or loud music is between 80 and 129 dB. As another point of reference: A jet engine is about 180 dB. A hearing test also measures the pitch or tone of what you're able to hear, and this provides more relevant information about the health of your hearing. For example, if the quietest sound you can hear is about 25 dB, that would be considered mild hearing loss.

Pure-Tone Hearing Test Results

Normal (-10–25)

Mild Hearing Loss (26–40)

Moderate Hearing Loss (41–55)

Moderately Severe Hearing Loss (56–70)

Severe Hearing Loss (70–90)

Profound Hearing Loss (91 or more)

Source: National Library of Medicine, National Center for Biotechnology Information

PELVIC EXAM/PAP SMEAR/HPV

A pelvic exam is an important part of a woman's regular OB-GYN checkup. It involves an assessment of various body parts including but not limited to the cervix, ovaries, rectum, uterus, vagina, and vulva. The frequency of pelvic exams will be based on several factors that need to be discussed with your healthcare provider.

WOMEN'S AGE (YEARS)	RECOMMENDATION*
21 to 29	• Pap test alone every 3 years • HPV testing alone can be considered, but Pap tests are preferred
30 to 65	• Option 1: Pap test and HPV test every 5 years (if previous results were within the standard range) • Option 2: Pap test alone every 3 years • Option 3: HPV testing alone every 5 years
65+	• No cervical cancer screening *if* you have never had abnormal cervical cells or cervical cancer, *and* you've had 2 or 3 negative screening tests in a row, depending on the type of test

Source: American College of Obstetrics and Gynecology

*Exceptions to guidelines that might call for more frequent screenings: history of cervical cancer, HIV positive, a weakened immune system, exposure before birth to diethylstilbestrol (DES)—a hormone given to pregnant women between 1940 and 1971.

A Pap smear is often part of this exam, which involves using a small, brushlike instrument to collect cells from the cervix that are analyzed to test for cervical cancer. This test can detect changes in cells that are not cancerous but are suggestive of cancer potentially developing in the future.

Certain types of human papillomavirus (HPV) can cause cervical cancer, so screening for it is important. HPV is the most common sexually transmitted disease and is readily spread by sexually active people of all ages engaging in unprotected sex. Many people will be infected by HPV at some point in their life but will be asymptomatic until years later when cancer develops. The good news is that in most cases, the virus will go away on its own without any need for treatment.

PROSTATE SCREENING/DIGITAL RECTAL EXAM (DRE)

There are two tests that doctors use to examine and assess the health of the prostate gland. The prostate-specific antigen (PSA) is a type of protein found in blood and semen. The PSA test is a blood test that measures the amount of this protein—high levels can indicate prostate cancer. The other test is the digital rectal exam, which is performed by the doctor inserting a gloved, lubricated finger into the rectum and feeling for any bumps or hardened areas that might be cancerous. This exam can be a little uncomfortable, but typically takes a short time and is not painful for most. In many cases, doctors recommend having both performed to give the most information about the health status of the prostate. Men at high risk (African Americans and other people of color, or those with one or more first-degree relatives with a history of prostate cancer at an early age, i.e., younger than 65) should start screening in their 40s. Talk to your doctor about this.

WHEN TO TALK TO YOUR DOCTOR BEFORE DECIDING ON TESTING

AGE	CIRCUMSTANCES
40	If you have more than one first-degree relative who had prostate cancer at an early age
45	For those at high risk
50	For men who are at average risk and expected to live 10 years or more

PROSTATE-SPECIFIC ANTIGEN (PSA) BLOOD TEST

RESULTS	STATUS
Less than 4 ng/ml	Normal
Between 4 and 10 ng/ml	Borderline (1 in 4 chance of having prostate cancer)
Greater than 10	Concerning (over 50 percent chance of having prostate cancer)

Source: American Cancer Society

SEXUALLY TRANSMITTED INFECTIONS (STIs)

People who are sexually active and engage in unprotected sex, especially with multiple partners or a single partner who has other relationships, should be vigilant about their STI status and get tested. STIs can often be silent without any symptoms, meaning you can be infected and not even know it. If you test positive for an STI, consider doing an additional test to confirm, then seek treatment from your healthcare provider. You'll also need to inform all your sexual partners, so they can be tested and treated as well, since infections can be transmitted back and forth. The type of STI testing you need as well as how often you should be screened depend on several variables including age, sexual behaviors, and other risk factors. Look at the chart on page 326 for some of the most common STIs.

INFECTION	TESTING RECOMMENDATIONS
Chlamydia and Gonorrhea	Sexually active women under age 25 Women older than age 25 and at increased risk of STIs—such as having unprotected sex with a new partner or multiple partners Men who have unprotected sex with men People with HIV Transgender women who have unprotected sex with men People who have been forced to have intercourse or engage in sexual activity against their will
Genital Herpes	It is generally recommended that testing be done only for people who have symptoms or other risk factors such as having a known contact with someone who has an infection. It's important to note that most people with herpes will never have any symptoms, but they can still spread the virus to others.
HIV/Syphilis/ Hepatitis	If you have any of the following risk factors, you should talk to your healthcare provider about testing: • Being pregnant or planning to become pregnant • Being forced to have intercourse or engage in sexual activity against your will • Having been in jail or prison • Having unprotected sex with more than one sexual partner, or if your partner has had multiple partners, since your last test • Intravenous (IV) drug use • Men who have unprotected sex with men • Newly diagnosed hepatitis C infection • Positive test for another STI, which puts you at greater risk of contracting other STIs • Symptoms of infection
HPV	• **Women:** between ages 25 and 65 should have an HPV test alone or an HPV test along with a Pap test every 5 years if previous test results were within the standard range. Those who are at high risk of cervical cancer or those who have irregular results on their Pap or HPV tests might have more frequent testing. • **Men:** regular testing isn't recommended, rather testing should be done for those who are experiencing symptoms such as genital warts

Source: Mayo Clinic

SKIN CHECK

Regardless of age, gender, or skin color, anyone can get skin cancer. It's true that people with fairer skin who spend a lot of time in the sun are at a much higher risk for skin cancer, but even those at lower risk (people with darker skin, people who've had less sun exposure) should be mindful of the condition of their skin and keep inventory of any changes that are seen. As many as one in five Americans will develop skin cancer in their lifetime, but the good news is that if it's caught early, it is highly treatable and the chances for a cure are greatly increased. One of the first lines of defense when it comes to preventing skin cancer is not just wearing the appropriate amount and type of sunscreen but also performing a skin self-check. No one sees your naked body more than you, so you are the best person to keep track of all the spots, rashes, and blemishes on your skin. It's critically important that you pay attention and note if these spots change in shape, color, size, and depth. If you notice any changes, make an appointment to see a dermatologist who will take a closer look.

To learn how to perform a skin self-exam, go to: https://youtube /UnCUcFJJDSA?si=g4S7iAX8VankkqAG.

URINALYSIS

A simple urine test can be like opening a large window into your health. Pee can be more than just that yellow fluid that fills the toilet and gets flushed away. Its color, smell, and what it contains can say a lot about how your kidneys are functioning, potential infections, cancer, and diabetes status. Doctors check if your urine contains blood, sugar, protein, and other things that might be an indicator of an underlying medical condition. Getting a urine test when you turn 30 is prudent, and even if it's normal, it gives you a baseline to compare it to future tests. Based on your results, further tests might be needed. Talk to your healthcare provider about how often you need this test.

The Inspiration

Kelly is a 53-year-old woman who had been neglecting her regular mammograms because of her busy schedule and an underlying fear. Despite knowing the importance of early detection, she had been postponing her screenings for several years. However, after noticing some unusual changes in her breast, she finally decided to undergo a mammogram.

During the mammogram, radiologists detected abnormal microcalcifications in Kelly's breast tissue. Following this, she underwent further tests, including a biopsy, which revealed ductal carcinoma in situ (DCIS), a very early stage of breast cancer where abnormal cells are found in the lining of a breast duct but have not spread outside the duct.

Upon diagnosis, Kelly was referred to an oncologist who discussed treatment options with her. Given the early stage of the cancer, her prognosis was very positive. The oncologist recommended a lumpectomy followed by radiation therapy to ensure complete removal of the abnormal cells and prevent recurrence.

The news of her diagnosis initially brought fear and anxiety for Kelly. However, with the support of her family and medical team, she found the strength to face her diagnosis head-on. Through education and counseling, she gained a better understanding of her condition and felt empowered to make informed decisions about her treatment.

Kelly underwent a successful lumpectomy, during which the abnormal cells were completely removed. She then completed a course of radiation therapy to target any remaining cancer cells and reduce the risk of recurrence. Throughout her treatment, Kelly experienced minimal side effects and was able to maintain her daily activities with the support of her loved ones.

The Change

Upon completion of treatment, Kelly's regular follow-up appointments showed no signs of cancer recurrence. She continued to prioritize her health, scheduling regular mammogram screenings and adopting a healthier lifestyle. Kelly's journey serves as a reminder of the importance of undergoing the appropriate exams in a timely manner as suggested by your healthcare provider. It's not uncommon for many people to experience fear and procrastination when it comes to healthcare screenings, but it's important to overcome these obstacles, because early detection, as in Kelly's case, can not only prevent unnecessary complications but can actually save your life.

10

YOUR TOP 10 NUMBERS

Numbers are important for assessing your health status. You might look fine and feel great on the outside, but there could be a completely different situation happening internally. Testing, measuring, imaging, analyzing, and diagnosing will inevitably involve numbers. What is blood pressure? What's the level of protein in the urine? What does the complete blood count show with regard to the hematocrit in a person who's complaining of shortness of breath? Healthcare professionals need numbers to refine and complete their assessments of most medical conditions. These numbers, however, are just not the purview of your healthcare provider. You also should know some important numbers and check them on a regular basis, as this will better inform you about what's going on or what might happen in the future.

This chapter is going to provide you with some extremely important numbers for each decade of your life. These might not be all the numbers you need to know, because you might have a health condition that requires you to monitor something differently. Use the list of numbers as a minimum guide to what you should know, but ask your healthcare provider if you need additional monitoring. For most people, these numbers are easy enough to measure either by your doctor or at home. The explanations offered in this section should make them easier to understand. Just like in the other chapters, feel free to look at other decades and consider some of those numbers that might

NUMBERS TO KNOW

30S	40S	50S	60S
Blood Glucose Levels	Blood Glucose Levels	Blood Glucose Levels	Blood Glucose Levels
Blood Pressure	Blood Pressure	Blood Pressure	Blood Pressure
Body Mass Index (BMI)	Calcium	Cholesterol	Cholesterol
Calcium	Cholesterol	Complete Blood Count	Complete Blood Count
Cholesterol	Complete Blood Count	Kidney Function	EKG
Complete Blood Count (CBC)	Kidney Function Tests	Mammogram (women)/ Prostate Specific Antigen (men)	Eye Pressure
STIs	Mammogram (women)/ Prostate Specific Antigen (men)	Prostate Specific Antigen (men)	Hearing Test
Triglycerides	Resting Heart Rate	Thyroid Function Tests	Kidney Function Tests
Urinalysis	Triglycerides	Triglycerides	Resting Heart Rate
Waist Circumference	Waist Circumference		Vitamin D

be different from what's listed in your decade. Most of these numbers can be obtained through simple, painless tests that are typically quick and easy to perform. Remember, the best patient is an informed patient, and that's exactly what this chapter aims to do.

30S

It's easy to think that given your youth and the many years ahead of you that your focus in your 30s wouldn't be on your health. You probably look and feel good, so why worry yourself about doctor appointments, tests, and numbers? You likely have more important concerns, such as career, family, social engagements, and building wealth. You'll start thinking about potential health dangers when you reach 50, a time when, according to popular belief, life suddenly changes. The truth, of course, is that life for most people doesn't suddenly change at 50. Rather, there are gradual changes occurring every year that accumulate undetected until a critical threshold is reached, and you begin experiencing the consequences of poor decisions and dismissing signs and symptoms as insignificant. This is the decade to be proactive and not sit by for the next decade or two when you might find yourself in a position where you must be reactive.

40S

This is a decade of change. You might be starting a new family or have already started one and your children are growing. You might be settled in a career or looking to venture off and try something different. Other interests have possibly kept you less engaged in your physical well-being and your health, and so you may have a few extra pounds around the midsection and face. Wrinkles are making an unwanted appearance, and your hair might be changing not only in color but also volume. A lot is happening at once, which can be confusing and frustrating and prompting you to look for answers.

50S

This is the decade to make a difference. In your 50s you can decide your life's path going forward and commit to making smart decisions and better choices that lead to optimal health. In this decade you can expect significant changes in your body, but they don't have to be all bad. You have the ability to make improvements, delay the onset of health challenges, and put yourself in a position to maintain a life of high-level functioning, whether it be in the gym, at work, or interacting with family and friends at home. There's no need to be anxious about what this decade might present if you are dialed in and in touch with your body. This self-awareness starts with finding out your numbers. Don't be afraid of this knowledge; rather, embrace it, store it, and use it to propel yourself to a better, healthier, and happier life.

60s+

This is an exciting decade and an opportunity to look forward to many more happy and productive years. Two of the most important things about the 60s are your attitude and your actions. Keeping yourself in a positive frame of mind is essential as you look back on what has happened in your life and look forward to all the life you have left to live. It's easy to fall into the trap of thinking that you're getting old and your time is limited and your body is going to start breaking down. That is absolutely not the perspective you want or need to put yourself in the position to squeeze the most out of life. Yes, as we age, there will be challenges and health setbacks and our body will not perform as it did in our younger years, but that absolutely does not mean you are sitting around passively and letting the years slip by as your body and mind deteriorate. This is a time to renew your dedication to life, become more robust, and challenge yourself both mentally and physically. Commit yourself to being proactive about your health. Rather than resigning yourself to a medical fate or ignoring symptoms, take the initiative to stay dialed in to your body, what you're experiencing, and what it all means. Knowing your numbers in critical health areas can go a long way in keeping your mind and body vigorous and capable. The next section contains the important numbers you need to know, but feel free to add to the list. Also, make sure you look at the 50s column in the Numbers to Know chart, and if you have never had any of those tests or haven't had them in the last 5 years, now might be a good time to get tested again. Remember, knowledge is power.

BLOOD PRESSURE

Our blood travels throughout our circulatory system, which includes our heart, arteries, veins, and capillaries. Blood pressure is defined as the amount of force the blood uses to get through the arteries. Imagine water going through a hose. There must be a certain amount of force to get the water through the hose and out the other end. The heart takes blood that is saturated with oxygen and pumps it out to the arteries. The arteries then deliver the oxygen-rich blood to the body's cells and tissues, where the oxygen is then offloaded and used for many purposes, including the all-important production of energy. When blood pressure is too high, it can be dangerous because the constant high pressure the blood exerts against the inside lining of the blood vessel walls can damage cells and tissues. This damage can lead to the accumulation of plaque; when it clumps too much, it starts narrowing the opening of the blood vessel, thus making it difficult for blood to flow through it. Less blood flow means diminished delivery of oxygen and other nutrients to the body's organs and tissues, and this can be extremely detrimental, in some cases leading to a heart attack or stroke. Conversely, blood pressure that is too low is also dangerous, because that means the pressure inside of the blood vessel is too weak to sustain a strong flow of blood. As in the case of high blood pressure, if the heart and blood vessels don't get enough blood to the target organs and tissues, they are deprived of vital oxygen and other nutrients. Measuring your blood pressure is the only way to know with certainty whether it's normal, too low, or too high.

BLOOD PRESSURE CATEGORY	SYSTOLIC MM HG (UPPER NUMBER)	AND/OR	DIASTOLIC MM HG (LOWER NUMBER)
Normal	Less than 120	and	Less than 80
Elevated	120 to 129	and	Less than 80
High Blood Pressure (Hypertension) Stage 1	130 to 139	or	80 to 89
High Blood Pressure (Hypertension) Stage 2	140 or Higher	or	90 or Higher
Hypertensive Crisis (consult your doctor immediately	Higher than 180	and/or	Higher than 120

Source: American Heart Association

BLOOD GLUCOSE (SUGAR) LEVELS

Glucose is the body's primary source of energy and is derived from the foods and beverages we consume. Blood glucose levels indicate the concentration of glucose in the bloodstream. It's important that we know this number as it can be predictive of imminent medical problems or the status of current health conditions.

BLOOD GLUCOSE (MILLIGRAMS PER DECILITER)

	FASTING	AFTER EATING
Normal	Less than 100	Less than 140
Prediabetes	100 to 126	140 to 200
Diabetes	Higher than 126	Higher than 200

Source: Adapted from American Diabetes Association

HEMOGLOBIN A1C (HBA1C) (%)

Normal	Less than 5.6
Prediabetes	5.7 to 6.4
Diabetes	Higher than 6.5

BODY MASS INDEX (BMI)

BMI is a measurement used to assess a person's body weight in relation to their height. This number is then used to categorize people into different weight categories. Full disclosure: Recently, the BMI chart and its inclusion in health analysis has come under fire. The first issue is that it was invented about 200 years ago and was exclusively based on white European males. Second, it didn't take into account that ethnicity, gender, and race can influence a person's body fat. BMI also varies according to people of different ages and their level of physical activity. Leading experts have not totally discounted the use of BMI to assess overall health and predict risk for diseases, but it should be just one of several tools in the toolbox. Other measures of risk that can be used in conjunction with BMI to help complete a health assessment are waist circumference, amount of visceral fat (fat located around abdominal organs), body composition (percentage of fat, bone, and muscles), and genetic factors. Your BMI is calculated by dividing your weight in pounds by your height in inches squared, then multiplied by 703. For example, if you are 5' 5" (65 inches) and weigh 145, your BMI is 24.1.

You can do this yourself or use an online calculator like the one found on the National Institutes of Health website: https://www.nhlbi.nih.gov/health/educational/lose_wt/BMI/bmicalc.htm.

BMI Calculation Formula: weight (lb) × 703 [height (in)]^2

BMI WEIGHT CLASSIFICATION

BMI	NUTRITIONAL STATUS
Below 18.5	Underweight
18.5 to 24.9	Normal weight
25.0 to 29.9	Pre-Obesity
30.0 to 34.9	Obesity class I
35.0 to 39.9	Obesity class II
Above 40	Obesity class III

Source: World Health Organization

CALCIUM

Calcium is the most abundant mineral in the body. It is absorbed through the lining of our small intestine, which then enters the bloodstream that carries it to the cells and bones. Almost 98 percent of calcium is deposited in our bones. It also features prominently in our teeth and is found in other parts of the body including our skeletal muscles (biceps, triceps, quads, abs, chest, among others) and in the fluid outside of our cells. Calcium allows our body to move properly by keeping our tissues flexible, rigid, and strong. We can consume calcium in food as well as through supplements. The body does an excellent job of regulating calcium levels, but if there's not enough or too much, problems can arise, such as poor nerve function, poor muscle control, heart malfunction (hypercalcemia), bone loss/thinning, confusion, depression, irritability, and memory problems (hypocalcemia). Our calcium blood levels can be measured with a simple blood test.

DIAGNOSTIC CATEGORY	CALCIUM (MILLIGRAMS PER DECILITER)
Low (Hypocalcemia)	Less than 8.5
Normal	8.5 to 10.5
High (Hypercalcemia)	Higher than 10.5

Source: National Institutes of Health

Note: Normal values and reference ranges may vary between laboratories by as much as 0.5 mg/dl, so check the values in the laboratory that performs the analysis.

CHOLESTEROL

There are three important numbers you need to know when measuring cholesterol. There are two major types of cholesterol that give you these numbers. LDL (low-density lipoprotein) is often called the bad cholesterol, because too much of it in your blood can *increase*

CATEGORY	TOTAL CHOLESTEROL (MG/DL)	LDL CHOLESTEROL (MG/DL)	HDL CHOLESTEROL (MG/DL)
Heart-Healthy	Less than 200	Less than 100	Less than 60
At-Risk	200 to 239	100 to 159	40 to 59 (male) 50 to 59 (female)
Dangerous	Higher than 240	Higher than 160	Higher than 40 (male) Higher than 50 (female)

Source: National Institutes of Health

your risk for heart disease and stroke. HDL (high-density lipoprotein) is often called the good cholesterol because high levels of it can help *lower* your risk for heart disease and stroke. Adding your LDL number and your HDL number gives you the total cholesterol number. All three—LDL, HDL, and total cholesterol—are important indicators of your risk for cardiovascular disease, so you need to know all three of them.

COMPLETE BLOOD COUNT (CBC)

The average human adult has more than 5 liters (6 quarts) of blood in their body. Without the proper amount of blood and the proper functioning of the various cell types within the blood, we simply can't live. The CBC is a simple blood test that is used to get a picture of a person's overall health and to look for the presence or risk of specific conditions such as anemia, infection, leukemia, and other bloodborne diseases. Health professionals look at the counts for particular cell types within the blood, and if they are found to be abnormal, this might help confirm a diagnosis or warrant further investigation to discover the underlying cause for the anomaly.

Human blood consists of three main categories of blood cells: red, white, and platelets. Red blood cells are the most common type. While they have many functions, the most important one is carrying oxygen throughout the body to all the cells, tissues, and organs that need it to function. Hemoglobin is the protein inside red blood cells that serves as a transporter by binding the oxygen as the blood circulates throughout the body.

White blood cells are the foot soldiers of the body's immune system. They travel throughout the blood until they get the signal that some part of the body is damaged. This damage could come in any form, but most likely it's something like a cut, infection, fracture, or allergic reaction. There are various types of white blood cells that look different and carry out different tasks; however, when needed, the different white blood cells team up in a coordinated fashion and fight the invading enemy in what is called an immune response. Not having enough white blood cells or having cells that are not working properly can cause significant problems. There are also conditions, such as leukemia, lymphoma, and sarcoidosis, when having too many white blood cells also creates health issues. This is why evaluating your white blood count periodically is important.

Platelets, also known as thrombocytes, are small, irregularly shaped, colorless cell fragments that circulate freely in the blood. When they are activated, they form clots and stop or help prevent bleeding. Not having enough platelets (thrombocytopenia) can be dangerous, because the body's ability to stop bleeding becomes impaired and could lead to dangerous levels of blood loss. Conversely, having too many platelets (thrombocythemia) is also a problem, because it can increase the risk of forming inappropriate blood clots that could deprive vital organs like the heart and brain of vital blood supply, potentially leading to heart attacks and strokes.

Your healthcare provider will compare your CBC results to a reference range of what is considered normal and assess whether there are areas that need to be addressed.

BLOOD COMPONENT	ABBREVIATION	REFERENCE RANGE
White Blood Cells	WBC	4,500 to 11,000/mm³
Red Blood Cells	RBC	Male: 4.3 to 5.9 million/mm³ Female: 3.5 to 5.5 million/mm³
Hemoglobin	HGB	Male: 13.5 to 17.5 g/dL Female: 12.0 to 16.0 g/dL
Hematocrit	HCT	Male: 41% to 53% Female: 36% to 46%
Mean Corpuscular Volume	MCV	80 to 100μm³
Mean Corpuscular Hemoglobin	MCH	25.4 to 34.6 pg/cell
Mean Corpuscular Hemoglobin Concentration	MCHC	31% to 36% Hb/cell
Platelets		150,000 to 4000,000/mm³

Source: National Center for Biotechnology Information

Note: Values differ depending on altitude. At higher altitudes (above 3,280 feet), hemoglobin and hematocrit will increase and this will be taken into consideration when your doctor analyzes the results.

ELECTROCARDIOGRAM (EKG)

The heart is a strong muscle that is powered by electrical activity that causes the four heart ventricles to contract. The condition of that electrical activity as well as the manner in which the heart beats are indicators of a normal heart or one that is not functioning properly. An electrocardiogram or EKG is a painless, noninvasive test in which electrodes are placed on various parts of the chest and limbs so they can record the electrical signals in the heart. A computer records this electrical activity and translates the information into a wave pattern that can be analyzed by a professional reading the results. Most people only need an EKG if they have symptoms, but getting an EKG even if you don't have any warning signs can be beneficial, because it gives you a baseline from which you can compare future EKGs. This can be valuable information for your doctor.

Symptoms That Might Lead to Needing an EKG

Chest pain

Dizziness/light-headedness/confusion

Fatigue (not explained by other causes)

Flutter or skipped heartbeat

Heart pounding

Rapid pulse

What an EKG Can Do

Assess heart rhythm for any abnormality (arrhythmia)

Assess how well certain heart disease treatments are working

Diagnose a heart attack

Diagnose an array of heart abnormalities (electrical activity, enlargement, valvular disease)

Diagnose heart failure

Diagnose heart muscle damage

Diagnose poor blood flow to the heart muscle due to coronary artery disease

Help assess a person's fitness for surgery

EYE PRESSURE

Our eyes are filled with fluid that allows them to function properly. This fluid, just like the blood in our blood vessels, exerts a force or pressure against the lining of our eyes. This pressure is called intra-ocular pressure, and the body regulates it automatically so that the eye has the best environment for good health. When the pressure is too high or too low, this could be dangerous to the eye and lead to impaired vision. Having an intraocular pressure that's too high and left untreated can damage the optic nerve, the all-important nerve that relays messages from the eyes to the brain to create visual images. A damaged optic nerve can lead not only to vision impairment, but if the damage is severe enough, it can lead to a total loss of vision. Glaucoma is a group of different eye conditions that damage the optic nerve. Glaucoma can happen even when the eye pressure is normal, but it typically happens when eye pressure is too high. Rates of glaucoma increase as we age, and Black, Latino, and Hispanic people have a much higher rate than white people. Eye pressure is measured by a simple test called tonometry in which a machine shoots a brief puff of air against your eye and then measures the movement of your eye's outer layer, the cornea. There's also another common test in which your eye is numbed by drops and then a special tool is pressed against the cornea and a measurement is taken.

Normal Intraocular Eye Pressure
10–20 mmHg

Source: American Academy of Ophthalmology

Dr. Ian's Tip

MAKE YOUR GUT HAPPY: EAT BACTERIA

Not all bacteria are bad for you. In fact, there are between 300 to 1,000 different species of bacteria that are living in your gut right now. These gut bacteria are collectively called the *gut microbiota*, and they are critical to our overall health. There is a constant fight in our gut between the good bacteria and the bad, and the body likes to keep a balance between the two. If this balance is thrown out of whack, it can lead to myriad digestive problems. Eat fermented foods like yogurt, kimchi, sauerkraut, and cheese, or drink it in kombucha or kefir. You can also get good bacteria from probiotic supplements. Make sure you're eating plenty of fiber as well, since that feeds the healthy gut bacteria.

HEARING TEST

As we age, hearing loss becomes more likely. Approximately 14 percent of people between the ages of 45 and 64 have some degree of hearing loss. For people 65 and older, this incidence of hearing loss increases to as much as 30 percent. Many experts recommend getting your hearing tested every 10 years up until the age of 50, then every 3 years after that. There are many causes for hearing loss, such as physical trauma, autoimmune disease, medication side effects, loud noises, tumors, among others, many of which can be treated if caught early enough and before too much damage is done. It's important not to ignore any hearing problems you may experience. Get examined by your healthcare provider to determine what the cause or causes might be and what treatment options are available. A hearing test is painless and takes approximately 30 minutes. The most common one is the pure-tone hearing test, in which you wear headphones and the tester pushes buttons on a machine called the audiometer, which generates and presents pure tones at specific frequencies and volume levels through the headphones. The tester records the softest or least audible sound that the patient can hear. The loudness of sound is measured in decibels (dB). For example, a whisper is about 20 to 30 dB, whereas shouting or loud music is 80 to 129 dB. As another point of reference, a jet engine is about 180 dB. A hearing test also measures the pitch or tone of what you're able to hear, and this provides more relevant information about the health of your hearing. For example, if the quietest sound you can hear is about 25 dB, that would be considered mild hearing loss.

Pure-Tone Hearing Test Results

Normal (-10–25)

Mild hearing loss (26–40)

Moderate hearing loss
(41–55)

Moderately severe hearing
loss (56–70)

Severe hearing loss
(70–90)

Profound hearing loss
(91 or more)

Source: National Library of Medicine, National Center for Biotechnology Information

KIDNEY FUNCTION TESTS

People over the age of 65 are at an increased risk of kidney diseases. Black, Latino, and Hispanic people as well as American Indians have an increased risk for developing kidney disease. One of the most important functions of the kidneys is to filter the blood by removing cellular waste and excess water by making urine, which is eventually eliminated through the urinary tract and out of the body. Kidney function tests are urine or blood tests that assess how well the kidneys are doing their job of cleaning the blood. The most common kidney function tests follow.

BLOOD UREA NITROGEN (BUN)

Urea nitrogen is a waste product that is formed when the body breaks down the protein we consume in foods. Urea nitrogen forms in the liver and is transported through the blood to the kidneys, where it's filtered out of the blood and travels out of the body in our urine. It's normal to have a small amount of urea nitrogen in the blood, but if there's too much, that's an indication that the kidneys are not working properly.

Blood Urea Nitrogen (BUN)
Normal: 5–20 mg/dL

CREATININE

When the body digests the protein in food, it creates a waste product called creatinine. This compound is also formed during the process of normal breakdown of muscle tissue. The kidneys clear creatinine from the blood and excrete it through the urine. Having too much creatinine in your urine could be an indication that there is a kidney problem. A creatinine test in conjunction with other tests, such as BUN and glomerular filtration rate (GFR), can help give a clearer picture of the kidneys' health and how well they are functioning.

CREATININE

GENDER	CREATININE (MILLIGRAMS PER DECILITER)
Adult Women	0.59 to 1.04
Adult Men	0.74 to 1.35

Source: Mayo Clinic

GLOMERULAR FILTRATION RATE (GFR)

As the kidneys are removing waste from the blood, they do so at a particular rate called the glomerular filtration rate (GFR). This rate shows how well the kidneys are doing their job of filtering waste products.

GLOMERULAR FILTRATION RATE (GFR)

GFR	CLASSIFICATION
60 or greater	Normal
Less than 60	Possible kidney disease
15 or lower	Possible kidney failure

URINE ALBUMIN

This is a protein that is produced in the liver and circulates in the blood as well as other bodily fluids such as urine. It's the most common type of protein in the blood and helps move enzymes, hormones, and nutrients through the body. Large amounts of albumin outside of the blood can indicate a problem. When kidneys are healthy, they don't allow albumin to pass from the blood into the urine. When a kidney is damaged and not functioning properly, it allows some albumin to slip through its cells and pass into the urine. Albuminuria is the term used to describe the presence of too much albumin in the urine.

URINE ALBUMIN

URINE ALBUMIN LEVEL	CLASSIFICATION
Below 30	Normal
Above 30	Possible kidney disease

MAMMOGRAM

The mammogram is a special X-ray imaging study of the breast to look for early signs of breast cancer. If these studies are performed adequately and regularly as recommended by your physician, breast cancer can be detected as much as 3 years earlier than it can actually be felt as a lump. The classification of results has been standardized by the Breast Imaging Reporting and Data System or BI-RADS. Always check with your doctor to determine when and how often you should undergo a mammogram screening test. You can learn more about mammograms in chapter 9.

MAMMOGRAM BI-RADS CATEGORIES

CATEGORY	DEFINITION	WHAT IT MEANS
0	Incomplete, additional imaging evaluation and/or comparison to prior mammograms (or other imaging tests) is needed.	The radiologist may have seen a possible abnormality, but it was unclear and you will need more tests, such as another mammogram with the use of spot compression (applying compression to a smaller area when doing the mammogram), magnified views, special mammogram views, and/or ultrasound. This may also suggest that the radiologist wants to compare your new mammogram with older ones to see if there have been changes in the area over time.
1	Negative	This is a normal test result. Your breasts look the same (they are symmetrical) with no masses (lumps), distorted structures, or suspicious calcifications. In this case, negative means nothing new or abnormal was found.
2	Benign (noncancerous) finding	This is also a negative test result (there's no sign of cancer), but the radiologist chooses to describe a finding that is not cancer, such as benign calcifications, masses, or lymph nodes in the breast. This can also be used to describe changes from a prior procedure (such as a biopsy) in the breast. This ensures that others who look at the mammogram in the future will not misinterpret the benign finding as suspicious.

| 3 | Probably benign finding. Follow-up in a short time frame is suggested. | A finding in this category has a very low (no more than 2%) chance of being cancer. It is not expected to change over time. But since it's not proven to be benign, it's helpful to be extra safe and see if the area in question does change over time. You will likely need follow-up with repeat imaging in 6 to 12 months and regularly after that until the finding is known to be stable (usually at least 2 years). This approach helps avoid unnecessary biopsies, but if the area does change over time, it still allows for early diagnosis. |
| 4 | Suspicious abnormality– Biopsy should be considered. | These findings do not definitely look like cancer but could be cancer. The radiologist is concerned enough to recommend a biopsy. The findings in this category can have a wide range of suspicion levels. For this reason, this category is often divided further: 4A: Finding with a low likelihood of being cancer (more than 2% but no more than 10%) 4B: Finding with a moderate likelihood of being cancer (more than 10% but no more than 50%) 4C: Finding with a high likelihood of being cancer (more than 50% but less than 95%), but not as high as Category 5. |

| 5 | Highly suggestive of malignancy. Appropriate action should be taken. | The findings look like cancer and have a high chance (at least 95%) of being cancer. Biopsy is very strongly recommended. |
| 6 | Known biopsy/proven malignancy. Appropriate action should be taken. | This category is only used for findings on a mammogram (or ultrasound or MRI) that have already been shown to be cancer by a previous biopsy. Imaging may be used in this way to see how well the cancer is responding to treatment. |

Source: American Cancer Society

PROSTATE-SPECIFIC ANTIGEN (PSA)

Prostate-specific antigen (PSA) is a protein produced by both normal *and* diseased cells of the prostate gland that's found only in men. The level of PSA in the blood in conjunction with other factors can indicate the likelihood there's a problem with your prostate, whether it be cancer, enlargement, or inflammation. The results of this simple blood test can help doctors not only diagnose disease but also keep track of the disease once diagnosed.

According to the National Cancer Institute, there is no specific normal or abnormal level of blood PSA. Whereas in the past, levels of 4.0 ng/mL were considered normal and unlikely to be a sign of prostate cancer, that thinking has changed. There are various factors that can make the PSA level increase and decrease that have nothing to do with cancer. There have been many cases in which a patient with a recorded PSA level of less still was diagnosed with cancer, as well as instances in which a high PSA level was recorded but no cancer was reported. This is why the PSA test should not be viewed as the only marker for prostate cancer but a suggestion to get further testing should the person's level, age, and medical history warrant it.

PSA TEST RESULTS

PSA (NG/ML)	CLASSIFICATION
Higher than 2.5	Abnormal
Less than 2.5	Normal
0.6 to 0.7	Median

Source: *Johns Hopkins Medicine*

Note: *These result classifications may vary with each person, so check with your doctor.*

RESTING HEART RATE

Our heart is a very thick muscle that is in alternating states of contraction and relaxation every second of our lives. There are times when our heart needs to beat faster (exercise) and times when our heart needs to beat slower (resting). In general terms, when the heart rate is lower at rest, it tends to be an indication of better heart function and good cardiovascular fitness. For example, well-trained athletes can get their heart rate up very high when they're exercising so they can meet their body's needs of delivering oxygen-rich blood to the body's tissues. However, when an athlete is resting and the demand for oxygen is much less, the heart doesn't beat anywhere near as fast, because it can do its job more efficiently.

One way to measure your pulse is to close your index and middle fingers together so there's no space between them, then place them on the side of your neck adjacent to your windpipe (trachea). You should be able to feel a pulse. That is your heartbeat. Look at your watch and count the number of beats for 15 seconds. Take that number and multiply it by 4; that will give you your heart rate in beats per minute.

Normal Resting Heart Rate
60 to 100 beats per min (bpm)

FACTORS INFLUENCING HEART RATE

- Age
- Air temperature
- Body position (sitting, standing up, lying down)

- Body size
- Emotions
- Fitness and activity levels
- Medical conditions (cardiovascular disease, diabetes, or high cholesterol)
- Medications
- Smoking

STIs

Unfortunately, sexually transmitted infections are more common than one might think, and according to the CDC many are on the rise compared to a decade ago. The statistics are daunting. One in 5 adults in the United States has an STI. More than 26 million new STIs occur each year, with half of them occurring in people aged 15 to 24 years old. These infections can start as something relatively benign, but if left undiagnosed and untreated, they can become seriously debilitating and annoying medical problems. There is also a financial public health impact as these infections cost a whopping $16 billion in direct medical costs each year. Many people are not even aware that they are infected, which is why vigilance is important. Using condoms, limiting the number of simultaneous sexual partners, and knowing your partner's sexual history are effective ways to limit transmission. It's unfortunate that many people associate shame with an STI diagnosis as this leads to the ignoring of symptoms and an unwillingness for those afflicted to seek a diagnosis and treatment. The 30s is often an extremely sexually active decade, which means that the likelihood of contracting an STI is greatly increased. The good news is that many of these STIs can be easily diagnosed with simple blood/fluid tests or small tissue samples. Even better news is that many of them are curable by medications, and if not cured, they can be managed well with the right treatment started in a timely manner. If you're at high risk (having had unprotected sex, for example), don't be embarrassed to ask your doctor to test you for an STI. It's better to be sure and to know the most you can about your sexual health so that you can lead a safe, productive, and enjoyable sex life.

Most Common STIs

Chlamydia	Human papillomavirus
Genital herpes	(HPV)
Gonorrhea	Syphilis
Hepatitis B	Trichomoniasis (Trich)
HIV	

Source: Centers for Disease Control and Prevention (CDC)

THYROID FUNCTION

The thyroid gland, a small, butterfly-shaped organ located in the front of the neck, makes the all-important thyroid hormone that is involved in numerous functions throughout the body such as energy usage (metabolism), weight regulation, hair growth, and temperature regulation. This hormone also keeps organs such as the heart and brain working optimally. Hyperthyroidism is a condition in which the body produces too much of the thyroid hormone. Conversely, hypothyroidism is when the body produces insufficient amounts of the hormone, which can lead to fatigue, weight gain, dry skin, muscle pain, constipation, and other problems.

There are two major forms of thyroid hormone: thyroxine (T4) and triiodothyronine (T3). T4 is the more abundant of the two circulating in the blood; however, to exert its effects properly in the body, it must be activated and converted into T3, a process that

THYROID FUNCTION TESTING NORMAL VALUES

HORMONE	HORMONE LEVEL
T4	5.0 to 12.0 µg/dL
T3	80 to 220 ng/dL
TSH	0.4 to 4.0 mIU/L

Source: American Thyroid Association

Note: These values are for a nonpregnant adult. These values can vary slightly according to the laboratory.

mainly occurs in the liver but also the gut, heart, muscles, and nerves.

The production of thyroid hormone is controlled by another hormone called the thyroid stimulating hormone (TSH), which is made by the pituitary gland located deep in the center of the brain. TSH stimulates the thyroid gland to produce thyroid hormone. When thyroid hormone levels are high or sufficient, the pituitary gland stops producing TSH; when thyroid hormone levels dip, the pituitary releases more TSH, causing the thyroid to produce more hormone. To assess the health of the thyroid gland and to find the cause of certain conditions, a blood test that measures the levels of T4, T3, and TSH can be extremely important.

TRIGLYCERIDES

Triglycerides are a type of fat that circulates with other lipids in our bloodstream. They are the most common type of fat in the body. There are two major ways we get triglycerides in our blood. First, we obtain them through the foods we eat (butter, oils, margarine, and other fats). Second, when our bodies don't burn all the calories in the food we consume, those extra calories get stored as triglycerides in our fat cells. The body does need some triglycerides for energy and function, however, having too many can be dangerous and lead to various conditions including heart and blood vessel disease. A simple

TRIGLYCERIDE LEVELS

CATEGORY	TRIGLYCERIDE (MG/DL)
Normal	<150
Borderline high	150 to 199
High	200 to 499
Very high	>500

Source: Johns Hopkins Medicine

blood test can measure the levels of triglycerides circulating in the bloodstream.

URINALYSIS

A urinalysis is a test that measures the microscopic contents found in the urine. This test can detect many conditions, including urinary tract infections (UTI), diabetes, and kidney problems. The major benefit of an occasional urinalysis is that it can detect signs of other problems such as kidney disease in the early stages. Getting a urinalysis at your annual checkup is easy and painless and can yield important information that can reveal a condition before symptoms appear. Remember, the best medicine starts with prevention.

VITAMIN D

Vitamin D is both a hormone and a nutrient. One of its most critical functions is to help the body absorb and retain calcium and phosphorus, two critical components for building bone and teeth. The immune system needs vitamin D to help combat infectious invasions from bacteria and viruses, muscles need it to move, and nerves need it to properly send signals.

Vitamin D can be found in some foods but very few that are naturally occurring. Most vitamin D is added to food—you might notice it on a label that says, "vitamin D fortified." Actually, one of the most important ways our body gets vitamin D is by making it, and that requires some help from the sun, which is why vitamin D is often referred to as the sunshine vitamin. Direct sunlight converts a chemical in the skin that begins the process of creating the active form of vitamin D, something called vitamin D_3 or calcitriol. People who don't get enough sunlight and don't eat enough foods containing vitamin D are at an increased risk of vitamin D deficiency, which might include bone pain, muscle weakness or aches, fatigue,

VITAMIN D STATUS

CLASSIFICATION	VITAMIN D (NG/ML)
Deficiency	Less than 20
Insufficient	21 to 29
Sufficient	Higher than 30
Intoxication (too high)	Higher than 150

Source: Holick M F. Vitamin D status: measurement, interpretation, and clinical application. Ann Epidemiol. 2009 Feb;19(2):73–8. doi: 10.1016/j.annepidem.2007.12.001. Epub 2008 Mar 10. PMID: 18329892; PMCID: PMC2665033.

or mood changes like depression. A blood test can detect whether you have a deficiency. It measures the level of 25-hydroxyvitamin D, also referred to as 25[OH]D. There are some differences of opinion on what the various levels mean, but the table above represents data from a consensus of experts. For more information about vitamin D, check out chapter 3.

WAIST CIRCUMFERENCE

Knowing your waist circumference is important, because it can be an indicator of whether you're at risk for heart disease, high blood pressure, high cholesterol, and type 2 diabetes. Waist circumference has been shown to be strongly associated with the risk of death regardless of one's BMI. Waist circumference is also one of the five criteria for metabolic syndrome, which is defined as having the presence of three or more of the following attributes: elevated fasting glucose, elevated triglycerides, hypertension (high blood pressure), large waist circumference, reduced HDL cholesterol. Waist circumference is also helpful when combined with body mass index (BMI). When those two measures are considered together, they provide stronger information as to whether a person is obese and at greater risk for health complications.

Measure your waist circumference by taking a tape measure and

HEALTHY WAIST CIRCUMFERENCE

Women	Less than 35 inches
Men	Less than 40 inches

starting at the top of your hip bone. Wrap it all the way around your body at the level of your belly button. The tape measure must be straight, even at the back, and not too tight. Despite the temptation to suck in your stomach and hold your breath as you measure, doing so will provide an inaccurate measurement. Record the number on the tape measure after you complete a full exhalation.

The Inspiration

Darius is a 45-year-old man who works as a project manager at a software development company. He leads a relatively active lifestyle, enjoying outdoor activities like hiking and cycling on weekends. Darius is health-conscious and pays attention to his diet, avoiding processed foods and prioritizing fruits, vegetables, and lean proteins. He doesn't smoke, and while he enjoys an occasional drink, he does so in moderation. Darius has a family history of hypertension, with his father being diagnosed with high blood pressure in his early 50s.

Over the past year, Darius has been monitoring his blood pressure regularly at home using a digital blood pressure monitor. He notices a slight increase in his readings, prompting him to schedule a visit with his primary care physician for further evaluation. His average readings have been consistently around 134/84 mmHg, which is slightly above the normal range.

Darius makes an appointment to see his doctor. During his visit, Darius's doctor conducts a comprehensive evaluation, including a review of his medical history, family history, and lifestyle factors. The doctor performs a physical examination and orders additional tests to assess Darius's overall health. While Darius's blood pressure isn't dangerously high, the upward trend raises concerns, especially given his family history.

The Plan

After careful evaluation, Darius's doctor recommends a multifaceted approach to managing his blood pressure:

Dietary modifications: The doctor advises Darius to further reduce his sodium intake and increase consumption of potassium-rich foods such as bananas, oranges, and leafy greens. Darius is also encouraged to maintain a diet rich in whole grains, lean proteins, and healthy fats like those found in avocados and nuts.

Regular exercise: Recognizing Darius's already active lifestyle, the doctor suggests incorporating more aerobic exercises, such as brisk walking or swimming, into his routine. Regular physical activity can help lower blood pressure and improve overall cardiovascular health.

Stress management: Stress can contribute to elevated blood pressure levels. Darius is encouraged to practice stress-reducing techniques such as mindfulness meditation, deep breathing exercises, and yoga to help manage his stress levels effectively.

Limiting alcohol intake: While Darius already drinks in moderation, the doctor advises him to further limit his alcohol consumption to no more than one drink per day.

Monitoring and follow-up: Darius is instructed to continue to regularly monitor his blood pressure at home and to keep track of his readings. He is scheduled for follow-up appointments to assess the effectiveness of the lifestyle modifications and make any necessary adjustments to his treatment plan.

The Change

Over the following months, Darius diligently follows the recommendations provided by his doctor. He adopts healthier dietary habits, engages in regular exercise, and incorporates stress-reducing activities into his daily routine. As a result, Darius's blood pressure gradually decreases, returning to within the normal range. He feels more energized, healthier, and confident in his ability to manage his blood pressure through lifestyle modifications. Darius's proactive approach to monitoring his health screening numbers has proven instrumental in identifying and addressing potential health concerns before they escalate.

NOTES

Chapter 1: Defy Age

1.   Y.E. Yegorov et al., "The Link between Chronic Stress and Accelerated Aging," *Biomedicines* 8, no. 7 (July 7, 2020): 198. doi:10.3390/biomedicines8070198.

2.   Z.M. Harvanek, et al., "Psychological and Biological Resilience Modulates the Effects of Stress on Epigenetic Aging," *Translational Psychiatry* 11, no. 1 (November 27, 2021): 601. https://doi.org/10.1038/s41398-021-01735-7.

Chapter 3: Your Top 10 Power Nutrients

1.   L.A. Tucker, "Dietary Fiber and Telomere Length in 5674 U.S. Adults: An NHANES Study of Biological Aging," *Nutrients*, 10, no. 4 (March 23, 2018): 400. doi: 10.3390/nu10040400. PMID: 29570620; PMCID: PMC5946185.

Chapter 8: The Body Fix

1.   Larry A. Tucker and Kayla Parker, "10-Year Weight Gain in 13,802 US Adults: The Role of Age, Sex, and Race," *Journal of Obesity* (May 6, 2022): 7652408. doi: 10.1155/2022/7652408.

2.   Ibid.

3.   Jodi L. Zilinski, et al., "Myocardial Adaptations to Recreational Marathon Training Among Middle-Aged Men," *Circulation: Cardiovascular Imaging*, 8, no. 2 (February 11, 2015): e002487. https://doi.org/10.1161/CIRCIMAGING.114.002487.

4.   Tucker and Parker, Ibid.

INDEX

NOTE: *Italic page references* indicate figures.